MONICA MAYHEM is originally from Brisbane, Queensland, and moved when she was 16 to Sydney, where she began a career in financial markets. She quit finance to become an exotic dancer at the Spearmint Rhino club, transitioning to hardcore porn after moving to Los Angeles in December 2000. She has since won many adult-industry awards, including the XRCO Starlet of the Year 2001, FOXE Vixen of the Year 2002 and KSEX Hottest Radio Babe 2006. She has also been inducted into the Hall of Fame at the Erotic Museum in Las Vegas. Over-18s can visit her website at www.monicamayhem.com.

GERRIE LIM was educated in Western Australia and Southern California, and met Monica Mayhem in 2001 when he interviewed her for *AVN Online*, the American adult-internet trade journal. At the time, he was based in Los Angeles as the 'Cinema Blue' columnist for *Penthouse Variations* magazine. He is the author of five previous books, most notably *In Lust We Trust: Adventures in Adult Cinema* and *Idol to Icon: The Creation of Celebrity Brands*.

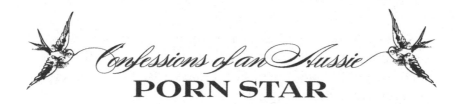

Confessions of an Aussie
PORN STAR

Absolute
MAYHEM

Monica Mayhem
Gerrie Lim

SKYHORSE PUBLISHING

Skyhorse Publishing books may be purchased in bulk at special discounts for sales promotion, corporate gifts, fund-raising, or educational purposes. Special editions can also be created to specifications. For details, contact the Special Sales Department, Skyhorse Publishing, 307 West 36th Street, 11th Floor, New York, NY 10018 or info@skyhorsepublishing.com.

www.skyhorsepublishing.com

10 9 8 7 6 5 4 3 2

Library of Congress Cataloging-in-Publication Data is available on file.

ISBN: 978-1-61608-091-4

Printed in the United States of America

To my cat, Smokey.
My ray of light in this dark world!

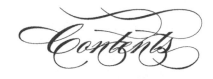

Contents

A DANGEROUS BUSINESS

Do you really want to know what it's like to be a porn star? Brace yourself, because I'm not going to pull any punches. Here's what a 'busy day at the office' might mean for me.

In September 2008, I did a video shoot in which we filmed three scenes in one day. When you're the star of the show, it's normal that you'll perform in three of its scenes, but shooting them all in one day is a big task. The shoot was organised by Robbye Bentley, a photographer friend of mine who had shot some of the very best of my early photos back in 2001, my first year in what we folks in porn jokingly call the 'jizz biz'. She had now turned director and was making a comeback in the industry after a few years off. We were on a tight budget, so I was going to have to work my ass off (not literally in this case, thankfully).

The first scene, in which I played opposite Tommy Gunn, was an office set-up in which we were two colleagues working late who decided to have some fun. Off-camera, we rubbed baby oil on each other's bodies so that we'd look all hot and sweaty, but this meant we found ourselves slipping and sliding everywhere. We tried to fuck on an office desk in the missionary position but we kept slipping off. The scene ended with us on the floor in the spoon position, but this meant I got a bunch of carpet-burns all over my body.

Then came the next scene, a girl–girl with the gorgeous Ava Rose, who has a nice big ass that I just love. The set-up was really cool: I was dressed like a total lesbian, in overalls and a wife-beater, with a bandana on my head, and I straight-up looked like I should have been on *The L Word*. We were working in a factory, by a conveyor belt, and Ava came in as my boss, dressed in a sexy little uniform and stilettos, telling me that I needed to work even more overtime. So I got pissed off and grabbed her and ripped open her dress, and we started fucking. This was difficult to shoot, though, because all we had to work with was the conveyor belt. We did some standing pussy-eating and then laid down some cardboard and went to town with the toys. It was a hot scene.

The third scene was a solo. By that stage, it was 9 pm, and we'd started the day at 9 am, so I was exhausted. Mercifully, we did have short breaks in between each scene, while the crew moved the furniture around, and these let us loose on the huge spread of food that was laid on (I get really hungry on shoots!). I managed to get a second wind right before the cameras rolled. It was the same factory set-up, only this time I was wearing a sexy bikini with cut-off denim shorts and strappy heels. I did a sexy striptease, then masturbation, including toys.

The way it was shot was beautiful: lots of close-ups of my face, my body, the hardcore action and, of course, the wide shots. I know, I'm getting very technical here, but these things make a huge difference to how a movie will look. Good lighting is key, too. The production team were great – they made sure everything was taken care of, and each set looked amazing.

Even though I had to pull a 13-hour day, it turned out really well and it was a great shoot. Pity that I don't know the name of the movie, or if it even came out. That's typical in porn, where a lot of movies get shot with no working titles and it's difficult to track them down later. Afterwards, I was so tired that I just went home. I took a hot bath, then lay in bed and watched TV. It was a long day, one of those days where you just head home and crash.

Sure, it was hard work, but I've had a lot of experience. I've been on this career path for over eight years now, and it's amazing to think that after turning 30 back in March 2008 I am still exposing my body for a living. Eight years is a really long time in the adult-film industry. The burnout rate in this business is brutal, and many girls don't even get past the first year. They quit, get lost in drugs or therapy, turn to full-time escort work or find something else to do. This is a US$12-billion industry that really runs like an incestuous little private club, where many are called and few really get chosen. And by chosen I mean make the cut, as in stay working longer than the first couple of years.

There are many, many things most people don't know about what it's really like being a porn star – such as how expensive it is. I paid US$6000 for my breast enhancements and still spend at least U$2000 a month on keeping up my appearance for the cameras and the fans. It breaks down to something like US$260 for my chiropractor, US$200 on hair, US$200 on nails, US$200 on acupuncture, US$110 on massages, US$140 on tanning, US$120 on STD tests, US$120 on facials, US$40 for the gym and the rest on constantly updating my wardrobe with clothes for shooting in and outfits for red-carpet events and nightclubs.

It's also a dangerous business. From potential STDs to living in a world where drug use happens openly every day, there are plenty of ways for a girl to get dragged down. You really need to erect a barrier between your true self and your professional persona, for your own protection. There is the 'sexy, mysterious porn star me' and then there is the 'regular me' outside of work. I compartmentalise. That's how you maintain your own standards, pertaining to what you will or won't do. And you have to do this all the time, every day.

So what am I still doing here, more than 400 movies later? Why am I still busting my hump for the viewing pleasure of millions who procure my good looks on DVD and the internet? Crudely put, I've pretty much sucked and fucked everyone I've been cast with (some of them multiple times and not always enjoyably so) and bared myself body and soul in more positions that I can even remember.

The basic answer to that question is the same one I tell reporters when they interview me. 'I just love getting fucked,' I tell them, and watch them try not to react. But there's more to it than that. Honestly, it's being desired that is my drug of choice. That's what I truly crave.

And if you really want the full answer, you should also remember this. The road to LA and my life as a porn star started for me when I was 14, living in suburban Brisbane, on the night I kicked my mum across the room.

Chapter One

MOTHER DEAREST

My dad shoving soap into my mouth for swearing – that's my earliest childhood memory, and I was only three years old. If that sounds weird, consider the next thing I remember after that: masturbating when I was five.

And it all went downhill from there.

I was born in Brisbane in the suburb of Brookfield, in the district of Moggill, some ten kilometres west of Brisbane city proper. It was a conservative suburb, with a small population but lots of land and some big Queenslander houses. There were places to go and ride horses and a farmer's market with locally grown fruit and vegetables, that type of thing.

My mother was born and raised in Wales. She had blue eyes, dark-brown hair, which she always kept short, and an olive complexion. When she was 19 and living in London, she jumped on a ship to Australia and ended up in Sydney. She met my dad in London, after moving back there from Sydney, which was an odd sort of parallel because my dad is actually from a coastal town in New South Wales a couple of hours north of Sydney. They got married in London and eventually made their way back to Australia, via Madrid, where my mother gave birth to my brother at the age of 30. Then, two years later, she gave birth to me in Brisbane.

My mother was six years older than my father and she was always bossing him around and putting him down. This was in spite of the fact that he was the breadwinner of the family – he worked in the music business as a recording engineer and radio DJ. Mum wasn't at all a big woman – she stood just five feet tall – but she certainly made up for her lack of physical stature with a quick temper and an angry disposition. She was an alcoholic, too. My father put up with it for seven years, for the sake of us kids, until my mother kicked him out in a fit of rage one night. They divorced when I was three years old.

At the time, we were living in Kenmore, adjacent to Brookfield. It was a good suburb, and after my dad left we clearly couldn't afford it. I remember a lot of hills, a lot of trees and a lot of really beautifully kept gardens. In the houses my mother rented, we had our own bedrooms, and some places even had a swimming pool. Kenmore was really my mother's way of keeping up with the Joneses – almost literally, since Jones is a very Welsh name!

After the divorce, my mother won custody of me and my brother (who has requested his name be withheld from this book), so we were left alone with her incessant smoking and drinking. She smoked Martin Blues – quite a rare brand, whose scarcity often made her settle for Benson & Hedges or Dunhills in the blue box. As for the booze, she drank the worst, most awful white wine – usually a Riesling or a sweet, fruity Lexia that came from a cask. Since it was cheap, and she was on the welfare, she would drink this crap all day and all night, and basically stayed drunk the whole time as her means of getting through life. She was also a serious pill popper. I don't recall a time when she wasn't hooked on pills. Don't ask me what they were, since I never checked the labels, but she had so many of them.

The remainder of her government welfare money she would spend on fine foods and other treats for herself, without ever thinking of me and my brother. On that account alone, I guess, anyone could consider her to have been selfish and cruel. But that was her nature. She was a very cold, bitter, aggressive woman.

She had this habit of always sitting outdoors – on the verandah or on the plastic patio furniture in the back yard – smoking and drinking and reading Stephen King novels. She would do this for hours, and you couldn't talk to her. Every time I tried, she would tell me to go piss off. And then she'd chain-smoke her cigs everywhere, even though she knew I was a chronic asthmatic, and whenever I started to choke and cough she'd just tell me to shut up.

In the mornings, she used to ring a bell from her bed and ask me to bring her tea or wine, often from as early as eleven. I was not allowed to sit down and talk to her until I had delivered it. Then she would watch old British comedies on TV – *The Benny Hill Show, Fawlty Towers* and *Monty Python*. Sometimes, I would watch them with her, and I grew to love them too. Mum seemed happier when she was watching these funny shows, and she was certainly less scary to be around. I tried so hard to get her to love me, and these seemed like the best times to be in her company.

She did work occasionally, but every time she got a secretarial job she would quit for some stupid reason – such as she didn't like the tea or she thought her boss was an asshole. She couldn't get on with anyone, really, and she didn't have many friends. The ones she did have, she ended up pushing away because of all the drama she brought into their lives, and people can only take so much. I only recall her ever having had two boyfriends after dad left. One was when I was five. Exactly who this guy was, I don't remember, but I know that he didn't last long. The other man was a Chinese scientist, whom she worked with in Brisbane. That was also short-term, only about a six-month relationship, because he ended up going back to China.

One of her good traits, which I inherited, was her cooking ability. She made amazing roasts and great Mediterranean food, although she was always smoking in the kitchen, so there must have been cigarette ashes in our food. And sometimes she got so drunk that she would forget that she'd already cooked dinner, and she would suddenly get up two hours later and cook another dinner, doing it all over again!

Did I complain? Of course not. She never gave me money for lunch at school so I was usually starving by the time I got home. I think this must have been why I was always so ridiculously skinny as a kid and why my brother and I sometimes stole a few dollars from her purse – just so we could eat. There was never anything in the fridge that I could take with me to school because she would always make sure to buy all this fancy shit that needed to be cooked and that only she could cook.

I went to Kenmore State School for primary school and absolutely hated the fact that I was the poorest kid there. We all had to wear school uniforms, so I was spared the embarrassment of people knowing my clothes outside school were all hand-me-downs from our neighbours' older daughters because my mum never took me shopping.

My school life was centred around a group of friends who, I'll admit, were not always the best kind. I was always putting some kind of gang together and became a bit of a problem child. I was a little smartass and got caned over the knuckles quite a few times.

But school wasn't always bad. One of my fondest early memories is of being six years old and choreographing little dance routines in the school courtyard with my friends at lunchtime. Most of the dances were to songs by Madonna, because her *Like a Virgin* album had just come out.

And then I put my first band together with a friend a couple of years older than me who played the keyboard. I could play the keyboard a bit myself, as well as the recorder, thanks to the occasional weekends when I'd got to visit my dad before he moved to Sydney that year. I'd never really kept it up, though, because my mother wouldn't pay for me to have lessons and didn't seem to want me to get into music – I guess because it reminded her of Dad. Anyway, in this band I sang and wrote the songs. (I don't remember many of them, because I threw most of them away.) I also joined the school choir – just for the chance to sing, and certainly not for the music itself since they made us sing such lame songs, mostly about Jesus, whom I didn't believe in.

The other area I excelled in was sports. My primary school was very sports-orientated, and I played tee-ball, softball and tennis. I was into little athletics and won a lot of competitions in the 100-metre sprints, hurdles and long jump. Amazingly, my mother would fork out for the after-school sports events. I also swam, though it was very hard to race in swimming because of my chronic asthma. I'd nearly died from an attack when I was three. I kept having major attacks after that, up to the age of around 12, where I would have to miss days at school and be put on a nebuliser (an oxygen machine). My mother would take care of me in this regard, too, as she would set up the machine and get me to the doctor that we always saw. I think she was actually worried that I could die every time I got a really bad asthma attack.

In short, my early life was defined mostly by my immersion in music and sports, which remain my strongest interests in life to this day (aside from sex, of course!).

After leaving primary school and progressing to high school, my life was marked less by music and sports and more by my actual involvement with a real gang. (Yes, drum roll, applause!) Whereas the little gangs at primary school were meaningless – never lasting long or amounting to anything more than a bunch of kids to run amok with – this gang was more organised. It had an identity and a name, which was known to the authorities.

I became more rebellious than ever, and I was smoking and drinking at the age of 12. By 13, I was ditching school a lot and spending my time hanging out at the creek or in the bush with my friends, smoking weed from home-made bongs, each one exquisitely crafted from a small orange-juice bottle with a piece of someone's hose and some tin for a cone. I wore an under-cut hairstyle and I used to sew my school-uniform skirts into tight miniskirts because I hated the long, ugly pleats.

I became the sort of kid that most social workers would probably classify a juvenile delinquent. The Juvenile Aid Bureau in Queensland is where troubled teens are sent for mandatory counselling, and I ended up in there a few times during my first high-school years, mostly for doing drugs.

In class, I was always arguing with teachers about why I needed to learn certain things and I felt like they could never give me a proper answer. I always believed I had a right to ask such questions. All that crap we were taught in school has proved absolutely useless when applied to my life. I made the maths teacher so mad that as punishment I was often sent to do my maths in the deputy-principal's office. The deputy-principal reminded me of my mother, in that she was always putting people down, and I think she singled me out for especially mean treatment, having obviously seen the rebellious side of me. Needless to say, we fought a lot.

Interestingly, at high school I excelled in all the artistic and creative stuff – art, drama, English, music, home economics, metalwork and woodwork. I had pretty much already given up sports: I was way too busy getting stoned, smoking cigs and drinking like a fish.

There were lots of girls at the school who liked to say they were going to become actresses and models, and I was one of them. Most of these girls thought they were too hot to trot, though. They would put me down and say mean things to my face, teasing me about my big eyes. I tried to ignore them, but it made me feel like an outcast, even inside my own peer group. There was always this sheen of negative energy around me. I have a photo of me taken when I was 12, wearing a black Mötley Crüe T-shirt and a very short black skirt that showed off my long, bare legs – the kind of legs they call 'legs for days'. My mother wrote on the back of that photo, 'Guess who? Still wants to be a model!' It was good to know that my own mother rated my chances as highly as my so-called friends. As it turned out, I'm the only one I know of who achieved their dream – even if it was slightly in the extreme!

Maybe surprisingly for someone who later became a porn star, I wasn't a hit with the boys at school. I think this was probably because they didn't like the fact that I was too tough for most of them. Those were my gang years. Most of the girls I knew had older siblings who were in gangs, and I got in through knowing them. We would crash parties and get into fights, often running from the cops and finding ourselves wanted for vandalism. We'd get wasted a lot and go to nightclubs, able to get in because Brisbane bouncers often didn't ask for ID and I looked much older than I was.

As I grew up, my mother's drinking became more and more a major source of embarrassment for me, and she would often humiliate me in front of my friends. She would show up at our hangouts and start yelling at all of them, telling them to leave me alone. She would call their parents when she was drunk, crying and talking nonsense, and even called the parents of my enemies, which made it intolerable for me at school. I lost a lot of friends because of all that.

One night when I was 14, my mum allowed me to attend a party. She said it would be fine as long as I came home by 11 pm, so off I went. My drug-taking had moved on to speed, acid and magic mushrooms by this stage, but that night I didn't do any, as I knew I'd have to face my mother. Maybe I drank a little, at most.

I was waiting outside for a ride back at exactly 11 pm when a police car pulled up, and one of the cops asked for me by name. I was initially fearful and didn't want to let him know who I was, until he said, 'We're looking for her because her mother's been in an accident.' So I went, 'Oh, shit. Yeah, that's me!' And I jumped into the police car and they drove me home.

Apparently, my mother had decided to go out at 9 pm to look for me. But she was already quite drunk – she was six times over the legal limit, they said – and had ended up wrapping her car around a pole. I found her sitting out front with a bleeding nose and clutching a glass of wine!

'Where were you?' she yelled when she saw me.

To which I replied, 'You fucking drunk bitch. You said I could go if I was home by eleven!'

She said she didn't remember telling me that. Clearly, she'd blacked out again, like she tended to do pretty much every night.

I turned to the cops. 'You're just going to leave me here like this?' I said to them, in exasperation. 'Look at her! What the fuck is wrong with you people?'

To my amazement, the cops said, 'You know, we can arrest you for swearing.'

I was incredulous. This couldn't be happening. 'This is fucked up!' I yelled, and I went inside and locked myself in my room.

And as for my mother, all that happened was they suspended her driver's licence for two years.

From around the age of ten, I was always trying to stay with my friends' families or get myself into foster care but the people at the child-services places didn't really help at all, probably because I didn't have actual proof of child abuse. It was mainly psychological with my mum. It got physical as well, but it didn't usually leave much of a mark. She would dig her long nails into my arm and slap me and fling me around. The slaps had turned to punches as I'd got older, and she would call me lots of names – 'little slut' was one of them, thereby preparing me for my future career (gee, thanks, Mum!).

Once, she tried to take us along to family counselling, in order to sort out our family problems. This was really weird since she seemed to me to be the one most in need of counselling. It was her way of blaming everything on us kids, blaming us for making her life miserable. She also did her utmost to keep us away from our father, by throwing away all the letters he wrote to us and spending all his child-support money on herself, on her wine and her cigs and fancy gourmet foods for the fridge. One time, I found out that she had spent a large cheque from my father on going shopping for herself after she bragged about it to my best friend's mother and this woman had then told me. I really think she didn't want us around and was resentful of the fact that she was stuck with us.

It all finally came to a head one night in the school holidays when I was 14. I was fast asleep in my bed when she stormed into my bedroom in the middle of the night. She actually stopped to take off her glasses before she started punching me in the face. She was shouting at me, accusing me of doing heroin (which wasn't true at all; I've never ever done heroin), and that's when I decided I'd had enough. It was time for me to fight back.

She clearly hadn't remembered that I'd started taking kick-boxing lessons in my friend's garage. As she perched above me in my bed, trying to keep punching me, I kicked her clear across the room.

'That's it!' she screamed. 'I want you out of here!'

I ran blindly out of the house, into the middle of nowhere. I'd taken no possessions with me, and I had no money, no bank account and no job. After racing thirty minutes through the bush, I finally reached a friend's house, where I spent the night, and after that I roamed from place to place. I remember sleeping under a bus stop a couple of times after getting lost, probably after doing some acid or when I was too drunk or too stoned to know where the hell I was.

A couple of days after she'd thrown me out, my mother had put up a 'MISSING CHILD' notice at the local McDonald's, where my gang usually hung out. That was *so* embarrassing! I know she did that not because she really wanted me back but because she didn't want people to think of her as a bad mother. In the meantime, there I was, moving all around the area – I stayed with a friend's family for a couple of months but I just wasn't accustomed to living in a normal, respectful household and they ended up kicking me out. I then moved in with one of my gang members, since I never formally left the gang, and slept on the floor for a couple of weeks.

At this juncture, sex began to play its key role in my young life. I was definitely, by nature, promiscuous. I'd always wanted to kiss the boys in primary school, and I'd started flashing my small boobs to them when I was six. By the age of 11, I'd wanted to lose my virginity, but for some reason the boys didn't notice me until I turned 14. That was the age when I had sex for the first time, with some kid from school.

He was 16, and I didn't really like him, but we got wasted at a party and spontaneously agreed to have sex on the way home – jumping each other's bones in someone's front yard. After a while, I sort of came to my senses and realised what was going on and told him to stop. He got it over and done with very quickly, and then he went round the school the next Monday bragging about it. Such a typical macho guy thing. He told everyone that I was a good fuck!

Some girls might have cringed or cried, but my reaction to that was, 'Well, at least he didn't say I was bad, right?' It's funny to me that it never occurred to him to wonder whether *he* was any good, but I guess that's like most boys of his age – sex is a one-way street and you're only interested in the bragging rights. And the way I reacted to it is pretty revealing. Even at that age, I already had this instinctive way of accepting myself as a sex object, since I didn't mind being called a 'good fuck' at all – in fact, I was rather proud of it.

What bearing might that have had on the fact that I finally became a porn star? Hmm, let's see now. Well, I had sex with some guy I didn't really know or even particularly like and became this romanticised sex object to him. Pardon my frankness, but isn't that what I went on to be for eight years and counting? That first time probably set the trend for my future. (That and my alcoholic mother's wonderful influence, of course.)

It turned out that being kicked out of home finally got me expelled from school. After the holidays, I tried to enrol myself in year ten but they wouldn't let me. The deputy-principal told me, 'You're not welcome here. You have no legal guardian, so you can't come back to school.'

'That's fine by me, bitch,' I said to her. 'I don't want to be here anyway. Fuck you!'

I've since been told that her reason for expelling me was bullshit, but that wouldn't have bothered me even if I'd known. I walked out of there with the biggest smile on my face. I hated that school so much. It was nothing but hell for me every single day, which was why I often ditched classes for weeks at a time. Leaving at the end of year nine meant I'd only had two years of high school, because we start at year eight in Queensland.

I slept with quite a few guys between then and the age of 16 – at least five that I can remember. They were all older than me and I never really had a relationship with any of them. I was just being promiscuous – because I craved attention, I think. Having sex was my way of feeling desired and loved. That and the fact that I enjoyed it so much!

I was seeing a 22-year-old guy at one point, when I was 14 or 15. He worked in a boiler room, as a welder, and he had an accident at work. When he was in the hospital, I went to visit him with a bunch of friends.

He asked everyone to leave except me, and I ended up giving him a blow job under the sheets! He was pretty high on morphine at that point, so I don't know how he even got it up. However, it was cut short when we were busted – when everyone walked back in and joked, 'What's goin' on in here?'

About three months after leaving home, I found a more or less permanent place to stay. I met an older girl at a party and she allowed me to share her flat with her. She was 22 and already had two kids, who were a real nightmare to deal with, but we got along quite well at first. I think she thought I was 17 and a bit more mature than some of the other girls I was hanging round with.

But nature took its course after a year or so. My flatmate found out that I was fucking her ex-boyfriend, whom she considered the love of her life. The situation was untenable, since I was in love with him too and had been seeing him for most of that year, behind her back. She actually saw us together while we were having sex. She shouted at me 'That's it!' and walked away. After-wards, she had a friend come into my room and start beating me when I was sleeping, just like my mother did. And once again, with feeling, I was outta there. Again, in the middle of the night. Again, into the middle of nowhere. *Déjà vu!*

It might surprise some people to learn that when I was a teenage runaway I never fucked guys for shelter. I know of porn stars who did, just so they could get food to eat and a roof over their heads, back when they were homeless like me. What I did instead was work and make my own money to survive.

I started off as a 'tea and tidy' girl at a hair salon, and then I worked as a cashier at a Big Rooster restaurant (which then became a Red Rooster, when they were all bought up and had their names changed). One of the older girls I used to hang out with did 'promotions' for a living, strutting her stuff in the nightclubs and pubs, clad usually in lingerie or a bikini, and she told me how great the money was. She referred me to the owners of the company, who interviewed me and explained how it worked. I was offered a job and immediately took it.

It turned out that the job entailed going to different pubs, clubs and bars around Brisbane, wherever I was booked, and pretty much doing whatever the managers asked: wearing lingerie and walking around selling raffle tickets, or wearing a bikini and washing the car windows of their customers. I wasn't promoting anything, really, just selling raffle tickets so people could win prizes, such as free booze or free dinners.

I was a little uncomfortable about doing this for three main reasons. Firstly, even though I got away with it, I was so young and had to always pretend to be 18. Secondly, all these drunk (and much older) men would try to hit on me. And thirdly, I felt very vulnerable wearing only lingerie, with no security guys anywhere in sight.

The job didn't last long. I had to catch so many buses just to get to where I had to be every time, and I'd usually turn up late. One day, I was very late and had to put on this complicated corset by myself, which took forever. The guy just fired me on the job, without paying me, after I had already worked one hour for him, so I never went back to it.

In the short time that I'd been a promotions model, though, I found I'd got used to parading myself in various states of undress and become comfortable with showing my body. In fact, I'd started to like being looked at, even though the stares came from men who just wanted to ogle me and fantasise about what I might look like totally naked. That's why I see that job today as an important step in my career. I seriously don't think I could've made it later as a stripper in London, much less a porn star in Los Angeles, if I hadn't first done promotions.

It was also my first experience of my personal survival being inextricably tied to monetary gain. If being seen half-naked was what it took to grant me my financial independence, then so be it. What we all ultimately want is to accrue enough 'fuck you money' – to be rich enough to say 'fuck you' to projects and people we're not interested in. And for me, at that age, with no school qualifications, promotions modelling seemed like a very good way to go. When you've come from nothing, there's nowhere to go but up.

After so long in the adult-film business, I have learned that this is a very common theme in the lives of many of us porn stars. It can be a fantastic confidence booster if you're a young girl still learning to express yourself through your body, needing to regain your self-esteem after years of parental abuse.

I think I will always have insecurities that have arisen from the ways in which I felt abandoned and neglected, mostly by my own family and so-called friends during my formative years in Queensland, and for that reason alone I'm certain I will never, ever move back to Brisbane. It's a city that reminds me of a past I'd rather forget. But because of my last few years living in my home town, these days when someone whips out a camera and tells me to take my clothes off it's the easiest thing to do in the whole wide world. I always went out clubbing half-naked anyway. Kerry Cohen, in her lovely memoir *Loose Girl: A Memoir of Promiscuity*, wrote about how a boy once told her it was tough for guys because they have to work so hard to get laid, whereas all she needed to do was walk around bra-less. I know that feeling, because that's exactly what I did. The power a near-naked woman can have over a man, I know it well. And I find it so intoxicating!

When I was just turning 15, however, I decided to take a 'real job' – doing legal conveyancing for the property market in Brisbane. I think they hired me for my enthusiasm in the interview and because I was willing to learn on the job. The office was a mess when I started working there, so I got stuck into reorganising everything. The company was called Fox Conveyancing and I worked there for a year. It was so small that they even had me as a manager at one point. We were responsible for all the necessary legal searches before a person or a company purchases a house or a plot of land – you know, all that small stuff like the title deeds and issues pertaining to bankruptcy and water and transportation (such as ensuring that they're not going to build a freeway over your house!). That job was crucial because it helped me get used to a more regimented way of working, preparing me for the world of financial markets.

At the time, I didn't know what path my future career would take, but it was enough to know that I had options. Little did I realise that, some eight years later, the legal and financial stuff would be completely out the window and, from another city on the other side of the world, I would be doing unimaginably crazy things such as selling my own used underwear from my website!

Chapter Two

MY BRILLIANT CAREER

fter the colossal psychic debris from the fallout with my mother, I knew that finding my father was something I just had to do. I had pretty much lost one parent, after all, so what did I have to lose in trying to find the other? I knew it was not exactly going to be easy, but somehow I needed to reconnect with him. I think I also felt a sense of purpose, because there was so much he didn't know in all the time he'd been gone and I kind of wanted to set the record straight.

Although he left when I was three, I still had memories deep inside me from the time when we were all together as a family. He used to sing me Beatles songs when I was a baby, so I grew up remembering many of the words in the Lennon/McCartney canon. To this day, I still love the Beatles because their music reminds me of my father. I saw him as a good guy who really didn't deserve the cruelty I'd been told my mother had heaped upon him, particularly the way she used to put him down in front of other people.

I hadn't seen him since I was about ten or 12. He had a wife now, whom I'd met in the past and had liked. They'd gone to live and work in Spain, but now, in 1994, they were back in Sydney, and I decided I was going to move there myself.

When I managed to get hold of him on the phone, I told him all about my life and how things had turned out with my mother and everything. He asked me if I wanted to move in with him and my stepmother, so they could help me out with my life. Of course, I jumped at his offer.

Seeing him again was weird, because I felt like a stranger. We had never really got to talk to or see each other much after the break-up. And as hard as he and my stepmum tried to make me feel wanted, I was still a rebellious teenager and a really messed-up kid. I know they were frustrated that they couldn't even give me hugs, since I was always so stand-offish. They gave me a lot of advice, although I hated being told what to do. I found a way to deal with it – it was easier to just say 'I agree' instead of trying to argue with them about everything. This seemed to work like a charm.

It helped that I really liked being in Sydney, which is still the city I plan to live in someday after I'm done with my life in entertainment. Sydney is just so beautiful everywhere you go, and there's something different in every suburb. The city is absolutely amazing, so modern, with skyscrapers and colourful lights. Darling Harbour was a new area then, and I liked what it had to offer, with lots of clubs and restaurants on the water. And, of course, there's Sydney Harbour itself, with the Opera House and the Harbour Bridge. The beaches are also wonderful, and I even liked the inner-city suburbs with all their different ethnicities and fine-dining opportunities. Everything was just so cool in Sydney. Brisbane was so slow in comparison. No wonder I got up to so much trouble there!

Sydney was a terrific place for me to start what I hoped would be my 'brilliant career'; however, the only problem was that I still didn't know exactly what I wanted that career to be.

Dad was encouraging me to sign up with a temp agency, to get a job that would build on the office skills I had picked up in the conveyancing company in Brisbane, but I had always kept in the back of my mind the notion that one day I would somehow work in entertainment. So I took a catwalk and photo-shoot course and got some pictures together for my portfolio. I got a few jobs out of it, and I was even in the Miss New South Wales Beach Girl competition. I did a couple of fashion shows in the Sydney nightclubs, one for Dolce & Gabbana lingerie and the other for a swimsuit company. Meanwhile, I also signed up with the temp agency, and it was through them that my career in the financial markets got started.

I was placed in a position as a secretary's assistant at Westpac bank – an entry-level job doing menial tasks as a way of learning the ropes. My job was mostly about doing administration and running around town, picking up reports and other documents for the senior economist. Then I moved on to doing lots of typing (reports and forecasts that the senior economist had written), making phone calls and photocopying and distributing reports to the dealers. And then I did more running around town, picking up or delivering more reports!

The job was only supposed to be for two weeks, but after that my employers at Westpac were so impressed with me that they offered me a full-time job as an economics assistant. I was still only 16 at the time and they required that I at least have my year-ten certificate – which I didn't, of course, having been expelled from school. I told them I did, though, and they hired me. (Sometimes, you've got to tell white lies to get your foot in the door!)

It was exciting at the time, particularly the rush of the dealing room, but it's also an insane work environment. Westpac was a good start but it was sort of like boot camp for me. I was basically a shit-kicker, doing way more work than my actual job was meant to require, because one of the girls whom I worked for was so lazy that I ended up doing most of her work. I should've had her job, and in fact they did leave me to do it for a whole month at one point, after she resigned.

I handled everything beautifully but they thought I was too young to fill her role permanently, so they got someone else in. Well, hell hath no fury like a rookie scorned. I decided I needed more of a challenge and applied for a job doing foreign-exchange settlements at Lloyds Bank NZA. I went for the interview and, somewhat to my surprise, actually got the job!

To this day, I still think of my job at the pre-ABN AMRO Lloyds Bank as the most memorable of my financial-markets career. We were like one big happy family, up on the 47th floor of the Governor Phillip Tower in Sydney (which appears in a scene in the Keanu Reeves film *The Matrix*). It had the most beautiful view of Sydney Harbour, and the people there were all so cool. We'd all go out drinking and attend corporate dinners, and I made many good friends out of it.

But shortly after, Lloyds Bank was acquired by ABN AMRO, and I had no choice but to stay with them. We had to move to the ABN AMRO offices, and things suddenly changed. Their whole corporate culture was so alien to us and it became not much fun to work there any more, but we still managed to go out and have a good time.

After living with my dad and stepmum for a year, I moved out and was living in Manly. I had a room in a three-person share-house. My two housemates were nice, although we didn't hang out as friends. We all kind of did our own thing – went to work and went out separately after work – so I can't say I knew either of them particularly well.

I used to get up at 6 am every day just to go surfing before work. I paid for surfing lessons, that's how I learned, but it was probably the hardest thing I've ever done as a sport and I actually wasn't all that great at it. You need sheer persistence to keep getting out there and trying again every time you get slammed by a huge wave, which is bad enough in itself but might also involve getting hit by your board or being forced underwater and then struggling to resurface.

After surfing, I would catch the JetCat – an express catamaran that used to shuttle back and forth between Manly and Circular Quay – to get to work, which was a really nice way to start the day. Life was good.

In order to meet more people and try something new, I also did a course in bartending and got a part-time job at a pub called The Orient Hotel in The Rocks. I had a great time tossing bottles and glasses, and I practised when it was quiet. That wasn't often, though, because the place was usually packed and really rowdy, and there were lots of brawls there. It was so much fun. I did that for about six months, and looking back now I don't know how I ever managed to juggle it with working full-time at Lloyds. I was doing at least a few shifts at the Orient every week – mostly weekends, meaning from Thursday to Sunday. I would go straight from work and get changed at the bar, and then get straight on with the bartending. (Talk about being a workaholic!) It did turn out as a great way for me to make new friends, though.

On nights when I didn't have a shift at the bar straight after work, I would go clubbing with the people from my bartending job, and it was on one of those nights that I took Ecstasy for the first time. That same crazy night, I met my first Lebanese boyfriend and I thought I was in love (when it was the Ecstasy speaking, of course). I spent most of the night dancing on the podium in the club while I was high as a kite, and so I was a serious mess the next day. I was supposed to work at the bar right afterwards, but I actually quit the bar job that very day. I just wanted to go out and have a good time for a change and felt I didn't need the extra money.

After living in Manly for six months, I left to move to the city, because it was taking me too long to get to work and back, especially if I wanted to go out clubbing at night. I got myself a studio apartment on Elizabeth Street, within walking distance to work and the clubs of Oxford Street.

Over the next few months, my life was all about clubbing, especially with my friend Kristie, whom I'd met out partying one night. Kristie lived in Penshurst, south of the city, and she asked me to move in with her. I was getting a bit lonely and was happy to have new friends, so I moved. I didn't care that it was almost as far away as Manly, because now I had more people to go clubbing with, and we would all pile into the car and drive. We had some crazy times together, doing loads of drugs and hanging out with a group of Lebanese men (who generally tended to have nothing to do with the drugs themselves), including that first guy whom I'd met and become smitten with. It was then that a few bad things happened in my Sydney life.

One night, I had organised to meet up with a friend's ex-boyfriend who was a DJ and had all the Ecstasy connections. I'd never met him before but had heard he was a good-looking guy who drove a red Honda Prelude. I went out with another friend and we were dressed up to the nines, as you tend to be when you're clubbing on Oxford Street. I was wearing this white vinyl dress, which, I guess, might have looked a little hookerish. We were standing on a street off Oxford Street waiting for him, and he was running late. Suddenly, this guy pulled up on the other side of the street in a red Honda Prelude. He was not bad looking, but not hot either. He waved for me to come over.

I went across the street while my friend waited. I said his name aloud and he said, 'Yep!'

I got in the car, handed him the money and he took it. Then I asked, 'So, can I have the Es?'

To my surprise, he pulled out his cock and started jerking off. 'How about a blow job?' he growled.

I was shocked. 'I don't think so!' I said. He responded by getting rough with me, grabbing my hair, leading me to wonder what the fuck was going on. I'd given him the money already, so I said, 'No, get the fuck off me!'

I asked his name again, and this time he said, 'No. You were expecting a drug dealer, huh?'

I quickly jumped out of the car and stood behind it, as if I was memorising his licence plate. I think he was still jerking off at that point. I then ran back to his window and said, 'Give me my fucking money back!' He threw it at me and threatened to call the cops on me. And I said I could do the same to him. I was so shocked. I ran in my high-heeled boots and called the DJ and told him what had happened. We ended up having a great night anyway, but I was shaking for quite a while after that.

Another night, I got beaten by one of the Lebanese guys, another of my new friends' ex-boyfriends, simply for taking her out to a club after they had broken up. I ended up taking him to court, and it really was one of the more unfortunate episodes in my life – because it brought back negative feelings from my years of childhood abuse, all the memories that I had repressed.

The Lebanese ex-boyfriend was psychotically obsessed with my friend, and when they broke up she begged me to go out clubbing with her on Oxford Street, which was a fateful move. When he saw us walking out of a club, he came up and punched me straight in the face, right in front of the bouncers. I blacked out and fell to the ground, and the bouncers took him out back and sorted him out. When I came to, I looked awful. My nose was swollen and bleeding, and it hurt like hell.

We drove to the police station and they took some photos. I pressed charges, but that didn't deter him. He found us the next day and from then on he followed us everywhere for a while, even to the police station! He was such a cocky bastard – he would drive by the station and rev his engine, then reverse up and down the street. The cops finally decided to chase him but they never caught him.

When the case came to court, the idiot represented himself. His story changed five times and he tried to act like a lawyer (obviously having watched one too many TV law shows). When he actually questioned me on the stand, he tried to put words in my mouth, but the judge saw right through him. And his ex-girlfriend (who was, by then, no longer my friend) was so scared of this guy that she said she hadn't seen anything. She was looking down the whole time while testifying and the judge commented on her body language and didn't believe her either. Basically, the guy got a slap on the wrist (merely a AU$1000 fine) and a warning that if he came near me again he would end up in jail.

Afterwards, I had to see a psychologist because I was having bad nightmares and serious bouts of depression.

The image of him hitting me kept replaying itself in my head. The psychologist tried out this hypnotherapy technique on me called 'rapid eye movement desensitisation'. He had me close my eyes and call up the image in my head of being hit that night. When I opened my eyes, I would follow his finger as he moved it from side to side. We kept doing this over many treatments, until finally I could no longer bring up the image. It was like he had pushed it to the back of my mind so all those feelings disappeared. I can't believe that it actually worked.

I realised I had been going down a very dangerous path, partying too much, taking too many drugs and putting myself in dodgy situations. One of my good friends, who was the head of the FX (foreign exchange) trading desk at ABN AMRO, offered me a room in his awesome house in Drummoyne – free of charge! All I had to do was help clean. He loved to cook, so he would make the tastiest dinners for us. This guy used to crack me up every time I walked into the dealing room at work, and he always stuck up for me like an older brother (or perhaps a father figure). If any guys made rude comments about me, he would yell at them.

Living with him, I finally got off the drugs, took up kick-boxing again and saved a lot of money. He was like my best friend, and I would look forward to coming home after work and having great conversations with him. But several years later, he found out about my porn career and didn't really talk to me after that. Clearly, he was not happy to know that at all. The last I knew of his whereabouts he was living in Byron Bay and had married a hippie chick. I learned he has a daughter and is trading from home, which was always his dream. I'm happy for him, but it would be nice if we could still be friends.

After a year and a half at the newly merged ABN AMRO/Lloyds Bank, I was fed up with the strictures of the new office climate, so I went for an interview at CBA Futures, for a position in futures clearing, and they hired me. Futures clearing is basically when all the financial transactions, usually from the futures-broking department or trading-floor deals, get thoroughly checked and approved before being processed or settled.

I stayed at CBA for three and a half years, working my way up to become an assistant financial controller in futures broking and clearing. When I wasn't out partying with my work colleagues, I was kick-boxing five nights a week (which added-up to ten hours a week!) at Thunderlegs gym in Granville. I also did a couple of gigs as a ring-card girl at some fights, which is where I met a new boyfriend, who was a fighter. I was with him for about six months. I had quit partying by that stage, because, obviously, kick-boxing and doing drugs just don't mix.

All the time I was working in the financial markets, I was always studying other things, pursuing my other dreams. I took a class on modelling for commercials and they got me a big hair show on a huge stage in front of a massive audience. I enjoyed being up on that stage, and it confirmed to me that I loved showing myself off in front of people. The only downside was that my hair got thrashed – they had coloured it with so many different dyes that when they tried to straighten it they couldn't. It was totally fried. Three hair stylists from a top salon couldn't even tame it, so they did an updo on me.

I think I was quite clueless about modelling, and I didn't pick the best agencies to work with. I was rejected from some of the top places, since at five foot five I was too short: the minimum height for modelling was five foot eight.

Feeling dejected about my modelling career, I decided at the ripe old age of 18 to get my Higher School Certificate via correspondence. I worked on that for a couple of years and did really well with my grades. I finished year 11 and started to work on year 12, but I was already working full-time, with longer hours and bigger responsibilities, so I decided I couldn't handle the correspondence courses any more and, perhaps regrettably, I stopped.

I took other classes, in an effort to sustain my sense of purpose. These included a whole variety of things, such as voice lessons, singing, acting and modelling, but I always got distracted with working or partying. I took a course in Swedish massage and almost completed that, but the idiot who taught it was a pervert who kept trying to get us all to go topless so he could teach us how to massage the chest, with no towel covering or anything. I knew what he was up to and, strange as it might seem now, given what I do for a living, I refused to take my top off.

And I was the *only* one who refused. He claimed it was a requirement to get my certificate, so I said, 'Fuck you!' and walked out. I've since practised my massage techniques on many guys and have nothing but good reports, so I hope he's reading this now!

About a year later, I joined Nutrimetics, a cosmetics company that was kind of like Avon, and that led to a course in beauty and make-up. I learned all about facials, pedicures and make-up application, and I ended up selling cosmetics on the side, and doing really well out of it. I hosted quite a few parties where I would either do facials or make-up and it was fun for a while, but bugging people and suffering their frequent rejection in the search for a sale was not for me, so I eventually gave that up.

I took courses in small-business management and Italian, and graduated from both with flying colours. I spoke very good Italian, too. ('*Buongiorno. Che bella gionarta. Come stai?*') I learned to write a business plan and found an investor to start my own clothing store, but that plan fell by the wayside for reasons coming up in the next chapter.

While at CBA Futures, I also did a course in futures broking and trading. I can't believe I actually learned about bond formulas, since I'd been kicked out of maths class every day in high school for being a smartass! I discovered that I was really good at foreign-exchange and futures calculations, from just learning on the job.

But my Pisces nature always got in the way of my advancement. I was always ready for a good time, instead of slogging away at a job or anything else. One of the absolute highlights of my time in Sydney was when the United States Navy came to town. My girl-friends and I had a blast for six days straight, hooking up with the sailors with their sexy white uniforms and those accents, and they were so sweet, too. I even got to go on the USS *Independence*, and for a little while afterwards one of the sailors and I stayed in touch.

In my corporate-finance years, I did have three sexual encounters with co-workers (though only three in six years makes me fairly innocent, if I may so humbly declare) – and one of them took place right on top of my desk at the Lloyds Bank offices in the Governor Phillip Tower, after hours.

It sounds like the kind of thing that people read in the pages of *Penthouse Forum*, but it actually happened to me. I was out on the town, having drinks with my co-workers at one of the many inter-office functions we attended. We were all very drunk, and I ended up dancing pretty hot and heavy with this one guy I worked with, who sat at a desk very close to mine. We both had after-hours access to the office on the 47th floor, so after the party ended we went up to the office and ended up fucking on my desk. Sex *above* the city – it was so hot!

The next day when he came into work, he looked over and winked at me. We started seeing each other after that, but he decided to get back with his ex-girlfriend (I always seem to get the guys who are still stuck on their exes), which made things weird between us for a while. We didn't speak to each other, and then the separation became permanent when Lloyds Bank got taken over by ABN AMRO – a blessing in disguise as far as that relationship was concerned.

Prior to that, when I was 16 and working in the dealing room at Westpac, I'd hooked up with one of the traders there. I'd noticed him always looking at me. Well, all the guys looked, but I *knew* he was interested, because every time I was alone or at the copy machine he would find an excuse to come over and talk to me. He eventually asked me out and I said yes.

Alcohol, as usual, played a part. On a drunken night out, we found ourselves making out on the dance floor in some bar and then went back to his place to fuck. I dated him for a while but he wasn't really my type, so I broke it off. It turned out that he really cared for me, and I guess I broke his heart, which made it kind of awkward to go to work.

The other time was with one of my close co-workers at CBA Futures. We worked on the same desk, and he was about to leave to go to college in Canada so we had a farewell dinner and drinks for him. We ended up drinking a lot and getting intimate at the table, followed by some dirty dancing and a trip back to his place. I swear, this guy had the biggest cock I'd ever seen – even bigger than most male porn stars I've been with. (Yes, even bigger than Billy Glide!) I remember that well: I was very sore the next day, because we'd fucked all night. We remained friends after that but haven't spoken for years.

The odd thing, now that I think about it, is that almost all the guys I fucked had really big cocks. Maybe I was destined to be a porn star after all!

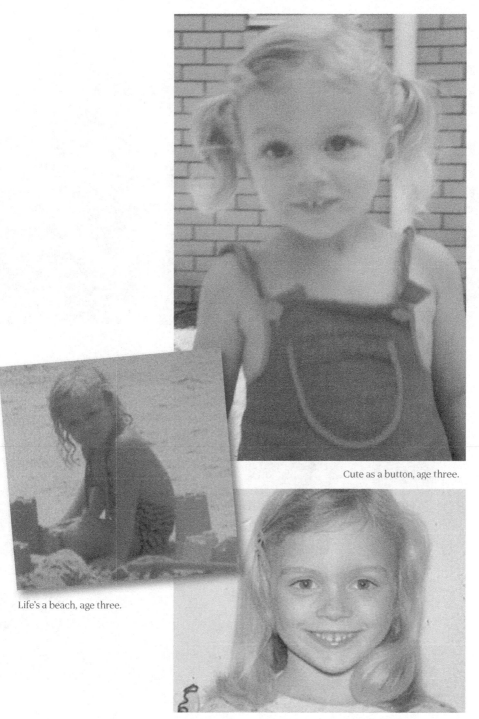

Cute as a button, age three.

Life's a beach, age three.

The future celebrity, age five.

Monica Mayhem

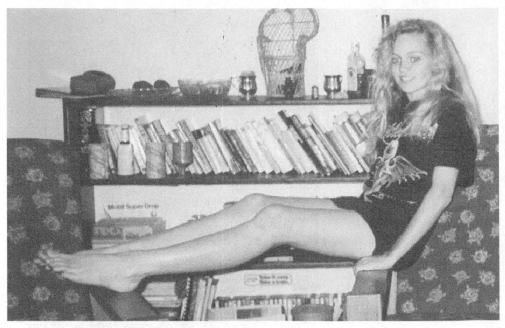

My Mötley Crüe T-shirt and 'legs for days', age 12.

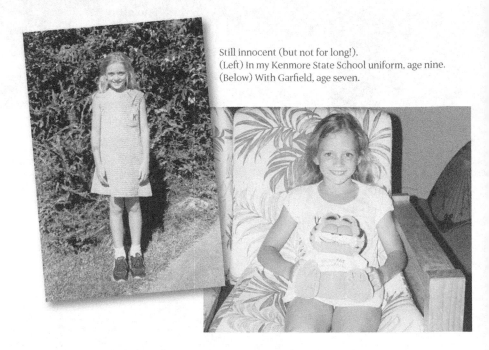

Still innocent (but not for long!).
(Left) In my Kenmore State School uniform, age nine.
(Below) With Garfield, age seven.

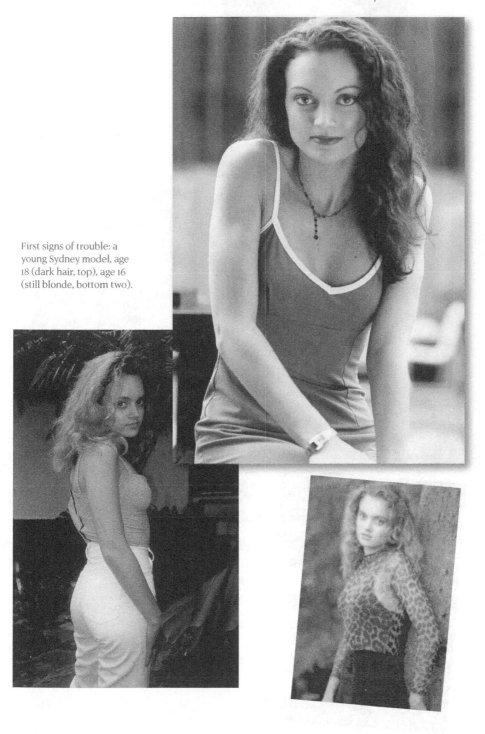

First signs of trouble: a young Sydney model, age 18 (dark hair, top), age 16 (still blonde, bottom two).

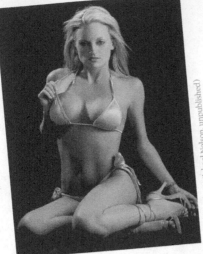

(Photo by Brett Michael Nelson. unpublished)

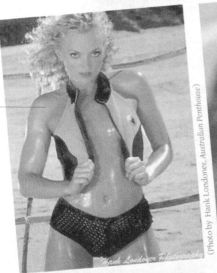

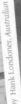

"Hank Londoner Photography"

(Photo by Hank Londoner. Australian Penthouse)

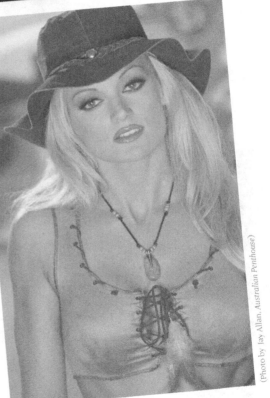

(Photo by Jay Allan. Australian Penthouse)

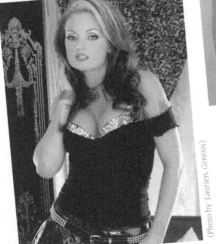

(Photo by Laurien. Genesis)

Life as a glamour/magazine model,
working my bod and bodice!

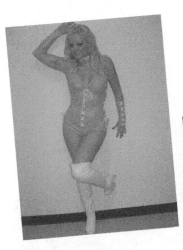

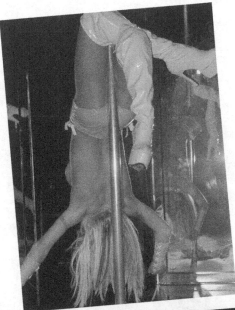

Life as a feature dancer,
working my pole
to get the guys'
poles working!

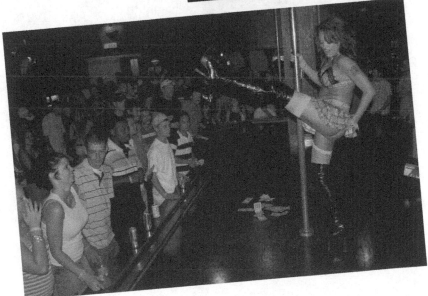

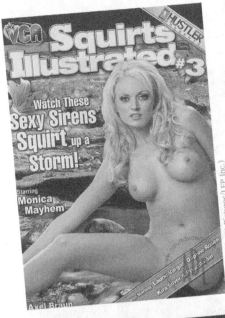

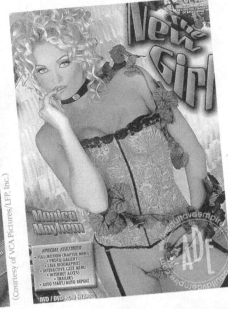

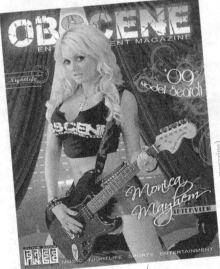

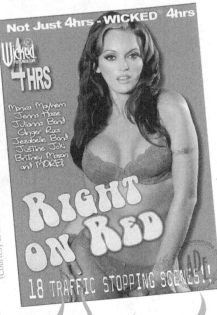

Some of my favourite movie and magazine covers!

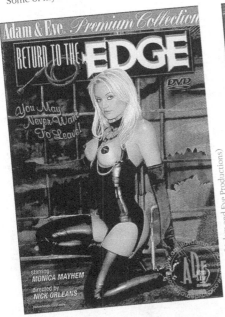

(Courtesy of Adam and Eve Productions)

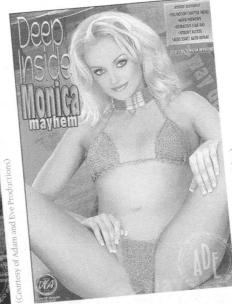

(Courtesy of VCA Pictures/LFP, Inc.)

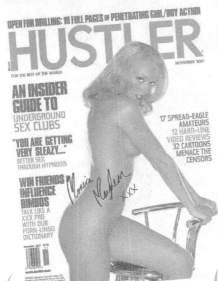

(Courtesy of Hustler/LFP, Inc.)

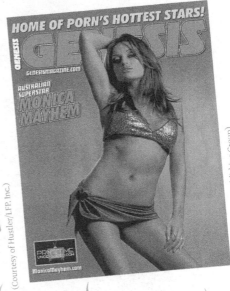

(Courtesy of Magna Publishing Group)

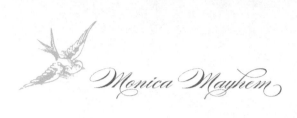

Monica Mayhem

Saucy enough for you? Photo shoot for my Saucy Aussie Collection of sex toys from Pipedream Products.

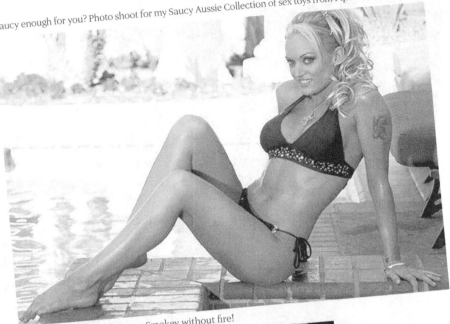

Me and my little healer – no Smokey without fire!

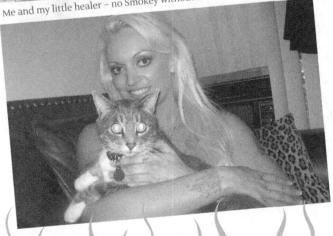

Chapter Three

LONDON CALLING

For my 21st birthday, my dad and stepmum gave me the amazing present of a return ticket to anywhere in the world I wanted to go. This was perfect for me because the travel bug had really hit me, and it forced me to save up the spending money and make it happen.

When I'd moved from Brisbane, all I'd wanted to do was see my dad, pick up the shattered pieces of my fractured family bonds and try to get a job so I could support myself and start a new life. I'd achieved all that now, and I'd had a great time in Sydney – mostly because of all the good friends I'd made – but it was time for a change.

I was so excited about the opportunity to leave Australia, and I saved up for a whole year to be able to afford a full European tour. I was always looking up the different trips I could take on the Contiki website. There were so many options. In the end, I chose one of those big Contiki bus tours that went to 12 countries in 37 days, starting and ending in London.

Arriving in London sure brought me back down to earth fast. When I got off the train from Heathrow, it was pouring with rain. I was carrying a huge backpack and had no idea where I was going. I remember that everyone was so rude. One guy was walking fast and got mad at me for walking slowly with my luggage. I was completely jet-lagged too, because I couldn't sleep at all on my 24-hour flight from Sydney.

It didn't take me too long to bounce back, though, and I set off for my European adventures in the esteemed company of 50 fellow Aussies, four Kiwis and two South Africans.

I cut down on my drinking during the tour, mostly because I really wanted to see Europe rather than merely partying my way through it. I didn't make many friends in that time as a result, but I saw a lot and actually remembered it all. I pretty much sampled every kind of food and alcoholic beverage there was (well, my new-found sobriety permitting) and kept an account of the trip in my journals. I wish I'd taken more photos. I shot mostly video and my camera died halfway through the trip, so most of what happened stayed firmly lodged in my own memories.

At first, I was treating these travels as no more than a great vacation, but somewhere on the trip I thought to myself, 'Well, what if I just work in London for a couple of years while I'm there? I could save some money and see where it takes me.' My Welsh roots made it an option, and the exchange rate at the time was about three to one, so any money I earned would be worth triple the amount in Australia. I guess, too, I was looking for some sort of escape. I was always trying to run away from something, which inevitably turned out to be myself.

When the tour ended and I got back to London, then, I moved in with my grandmother in Eltham. She was my mum's mum, and she was dying from breast cancer. Granddad had passed away years ago, and I'd only met them both twice, when they'd come to visit us in Australia. Now, I would have the chance to get to know my grandmother a bit better.

Being based in the UK meant I would also be able to visit my great-aunt and uncle and a bunch of cousins in Wales, whom I'd never met before. Despite my feelings about my mother, I have always identified very strongly with my Welsh heritage. Some of my relations were in the south, in Cardiff, and others way up north in Blaenau Fastening, Gwent (that's Blaenau Ffestiniog, Gwynedd, to the locals), where there's pretty much nothing around for miles but the slate mountains of Snowdonia.

I couldn't wait to see them and to see a bit of the country, so I headed over there after about a week in Eltham.

Sadly, it turned out to be very awkward meeting these relatives, because they were from my mother's side of the family and I got the feeling that they didn't really talk to her or know much about her. It was more that they were close to my grandmother.

When I was there, everyone spoke Welsh in front of me, knowing full well that I couldn't understand it, and it seemed that my cousins didn't care to get to know me. (After all, they were living up there compared with me growing up in Australia, so I suspect they were rather resentful of me!)

Being in northern Wales was a cool experience, though, because it seemed as if time had stood still. Today, Blaenau has a population of just under 5000 and is very dependent on tourism (thanks to the nearby Snowdonia National Park), since the slate-mining industry has been in decline for years.

I also travelled to Norwich in England, to see my aunt, my uncle and my cousins, who were all really cool people. My aunt, who is my mum's sister, was so nice and caring and polite, very sincere. It was amazing to see how she turned out, considering how my mother was.

Back in Eltham, I did my bit around the house by taking care of my grandmother, cleaning up and doing all the shopping and cooking. I sprayed ice on her sore muscles and helped her to get up and down the stairs. At the same time, I was very busy looking for work, visiting employment agencies and checking online and in the papers. I spent my free time making calls, attending interviews and going to internet cafes.

But it turned out that the things my mum had told me about my grandmother were true, and she was even crueller than my mother. It made me realise what a terrible time of it my mum must have had growing up with her. She would talk on the phone to her friends and relatives in Welsh, and I could tell from her tone that she was slagging me off. Every now and then she would break into English and I would overhear her saying that I was always on the phone and on the internet and that I wasn't working. (Well, I was trying to find a fucking job, that's why!) I couldn't believe she could do that, after all I did for her. Before even a month was up, she had kicked me out on the street.

In desperation, I got a job as a bartender in Hammersmith, but I lasted for only a week. I couldn't stand the 12-hour shifts with barely any breaks and I had to share a crappy little room with another girl. But then I was offered a job in International Petroleum Exchange (IPE) Broking at Salomon Smith Barney, and I told the bar manager I was giving him notice. He reacted by kicking me out too.

What the fuck was going on? It was a recurring pattern in my life – everyone seemed to leave me stranded!

Luckily, I had a friend from Australia, Mulvey, whom I used to work with at CBA. He was living in Putney, so he let me stay at his place for three months until I found somewhere of my own. He didn't charge me rent and even gave up his bedroom for me! (We're still friends today.)

My new job involved making sure that everything relating to the trades from the IPE were put through the system correctly and that all the transactions balanced out at the end of the day. Underneath the glamour of all that fast money being moved around, I honestly didn't have a good time at all at Salomon Smith Barney. The main reason was that the lady who was training me was a complete nightmare, and she couldn't explain anything properly. She was always very stressed out, usually over nothing, and would take twenty cigarette breaks a day. I hated working there. I'm sure a plum job at Salomon Smith Barney sounds great to most people, but I didn't last six months.

Some of the guys were cool, but several of them were sleazy. They talked among themselves, within my hearing, about how they could see my G-string. One of them even asked to buy my sweaty gym clothes, which really stunned me because he wasn't kidding. (I never sold them to him, in case you're wondering.) He was always making some kind of sexually suggestive remark about me and would talk to the other boys about what I was wearing that day. There were also times when he would get drunk and hit on me. I couldn't believe these guys! Back in Australia, it would have been the grounds for a sexual-harassment suit, but I didn't really know what the protocol was in the UK. I doubt I would have gone through with it anyhow, as I always prefer to sort my problems out myself.

There were so many things that I just didn't care for about London. Firstly, as everyone knows, there was the freezing-cold weather and the rain. I felt as if I could never get warm outside, and everywhere I went it was boiling hot inside, which was so ridiculous to an Aussie girl like me.

Secondly, there were the crowds – I couldn't move without someone bumping into me. This seemed to suit some people just fine, though, because I actually got felt up on the Tube by some guy in a business suit. It was rush hour, on the way to work, and the train was jam-packed. I was standing, holding on to a strap with one hand and my purse and umbrella with the other. I was dying of heat in my big coat, and the guy standing next to me – conveniently crushed in like the rest of us – said, 'It's like a pack of sardines, eh?'

I said, 'Yep.' And the next thing I knew, I felt his hand try to get around my umbrella and my purse. He wasn't interested in stealing my money; he was trying to get his hand under my coat!

I thought, well, it *is* kind of crowded and maybe I'm imagining things, so I moved a little to try to brush him off. But he kept doing it. I elbowed him really hard but it didn't stop him and I didn't know what to do. He still kept on and I kept trying to move away but there was nowhere to go. Finally, the train stopped and I pushed my way through the crowd. I got off at whatever station it was – I didn't care! I was totally freaked out. I couldn't believe what had just happened. Ever since then, I get panic attacks when I'm in crowds. We all drive in Los Angeles, so I can't even imagine catching a crowded train these days.

Then, thirdly, the food in London was just not to my liking. They heaped mayonnaise and cheese on every sandwich. I ate a lot of crap, except for the soups, which I loved, and the pub roasts, which were great. You can get a good meal if you have a lot of money to spend in a fancy restaurant, but there was little that was cheap and good. I did eat a lot of Indian food, which I thought was the best food in London. It was relatively affordable, too, and to this day I still absolutely love Indian food, although those creamy sauces are very fattening.

And that leads me to my fourth and final problem – the sheer cost of living in London, which was (and still is) absolutely outrageous. I don't know how anyone with a regular job can survive there. Everything, from rent to food, is so expensive! Why would anyone pay eight pounds for a plate of fish and chips or sludgy pasta that you can make yourself at home?

It was London that made me realise I was already so over the financial industry, and it was wearing me down and burning me out. It just wasn't what I wanted to do in the long run. I had always known it deep down, even when I was enjoying it more in Australia, but I never did anything about it because I was so comfortable with having all that money and all those benefits. When I was offered a higher position at Salomon Smith Barney, I found myself saying, 'You know what? I don't think I can handle it right now. This is not what I want to do.'

I had really found the space during those last months at Salomon Smith Barney to 'find myself' and decided that I still wanted to get involved somehow in the entertainment industry. So I quit.

I had already found myself a 'modelling' agent through the newspaper prior to this, when I was looking around to see what other kinds of work I could do. Being too short for a regular model, I'd gone for the other option: softcore. The agent had found me some paid work doing softcore photo shoots, and I'd taken him up on it. I also did a softcore-porn-film shoot that he'd booked me on for the Adult Channel with three other girls. It was a bit weird because I'd never been with a girl before, but we really didn't do much other than simulated pussy-eating. Getting naked wasn't too hard at that point either, after the photo shoots I'd done.

A lot of girls in adult entertainment get their start this way, getting half-naked for the cameraman before taking it all off for a live audience, and I wanted to see what that was like. I might've been insecure about many things but my body wasn't one of them.

Sure enough, I went from doing still- and video-camera poses to dancing nude on the chrome-pole stage. To this day, I can't remember the name of the club where I began stripping, but I didn't stay there long – it was just too far from where I was living. I don't even remember where it was located. I started there because it was the nicest club that I could find, and also because they took me in with no previous experience.

I became friends with another girl who stripped there – she was a very shy girl. When we heard that the Spearmint Rhino club was opening up in central London, we couldn't resist. I remember the first time I walked into the Spearmint Rhino, on Tottenham Court Road. It was so beautiful that I knew I wanted to work there.

I got the job by going in for an 'audition' – meaning I danced around the pole and got naked for them, so they could assess my competence. The Rhino was a 'long-gown' club, just like where I'd started. This meant we had to wear long, see-through gowns when we were walking the floor, rather than skimpy little outfits, because it looked more classy. It didn't take too long for the long gown to become no gown, of course, because the Rhino, also like my first club, was fully nude. Other things the two places had in common were that we didn't get to choose our own songs, and I always had to get a bit drunk before I could get up on stage. I wasn't ashamed of my body, but I still got nervous. Sometimes, I would also do a little blow.

When I started stripping, I didn't really know what I was doing, but I practised my moves when the club was empty and hung out with some of the other girls and got tips from them. I did enjoy the social elements of the job. When I wasn't on stage, I had to sit and chat and drink with the guys, which came very easily to me since I love to talk to new people, and I soon got the hang of it. Dancing naked for a bunch of Londoners: that does sound so strange after all those years in the financial markets, but the truth was that, for me, it was easy getting naked after a few drinks.

The best thing about dancing in London was all the rules. We had a six-foot rule (meaning the guys had to keep six feet away from us), so there were no dirty lap dances, as is common in the States. I was especially grateful for this when one of the guys from Salomon Smith Barney came into the Rhino to see me one night. I gave him a table dance, from six feet away, so he had no chance of groping me!

The money was pretty good, too. I could get paid £250 just to sit and have dinner and drinks with the customers for an hour. Some guys would pay me just to hang out and talk and drink with them. It was really fun, and I enjoyed being an entertainer on that very direct, personal level.

I never saw it as any kind of stepping stone, and getting into porn never crossed my mind at all. But in hindsight it was clearly an important transitional period in my life.

If I could go back in time, I would have stuck with the singing and acting classes that I'd started in Sydney and really tried to pursue that, rather than listen to what my parents wanted me to do. Their not encouraging me to pursue my dreams – well, that's still quite devastating to me. However, I think my life would have gone nowhere had I stayed at the Spearmint Rhino in London or just carried on as a glamour model doing softcore shoots. Looking back, I'm so glad I moved on. I didn't know then about half the things I was about to do (and might've shrieked in horror if I had known) but I'm certain that I would never have taken the time to go to mainstream acting auditions while I was stripping and doing glamour modelling in the UK.

After the madness of modelling for small-time photographers, shaking my booty for the lads and louts, and freezing my butt off while trying to analyse the volatile financial markets, I was ready for a serious change of lifestyle. London is a great place to visit but, personally, I couldn't handle living there. I was a fun-loving Aussie girl, and palm trees, pink sunsets, miles of beaches and throngs of beautiful people were much more my scene. Southern California was waiting for me.

So how did my big move from London to LA come about? It was simple: one night in December 2000 at the Spearmint Rhino, a bunch of us were getting drunk after work as usual when I dared one of the club's owners, an American, to fly me back to the States with him. To my complete astonishment, he called my bluff, and four hours later we were on a plane – I'd got a free trip to America!

I left everything behind and flew away on the wings of sheer spontaneity. I trusted my instincts to guide me onwards, even if most normal people would scarcely have considered it a good career move. My only plan at the time was to travel round the United States, hopefully making money by stripping, and then return to London to pick up the things that I'd left behind and take them and myself back to Sydney.

But things didn't quite turn out that way.

Chapter Four

LIKE A
VIRGIN

*A*fter doing more than 400 movies and magazine layouts, I find myself randomly remembering things I had once forgotten. Sequences of events come back to me in hazy flashes and sudden spurts, perhaps because I wasn't always entirely sober at the time (although I always am nowadays, as I'm much more conscious of my image).

This can be quite distracting when you take into account the outrageous, crazy or just downright ridiculous things I've experienced. One time, for instance, a bunch of us were smoking weed on set, and I was working with this guy who had really long balls. The camera couldn't see the hardcore action because of them. So the director yelled out, 'Hey, move your damn cow udders. I can't see the penetration.' I lost it after that, and we had to take a break. I was laughing so hard that tears were coming out of my eyes, and the make-up artist had to re-do my make-up!

Not being entirely sober on set is a common trait among quite a few porn stars, though we're not always allowed to admit it. In fact, we're not supposed to 'fess up to a lot of things. A producer I used to work with once threw a fit when she read one of my interviews in which I admitted that I have terrible trouble achieving orgasm from penetration, which is true and still remains my biggest problem sexually. But tsk, tsk, I was a porn star and porn stars don't say things like that! We're all supposed to be these super-orgasmic supersluts, don't you know?

Yep, my tough-Aussie swagger and my big mouth, those sure get me into all kinds of trouble. But I'd rather speak the truth instead of kowtowing to some prescribed standard that's hypocritical or false. And *that's* not something that's common to most porn stars, most of whom happily toe the line, doing what they're told. I have never been able to do that, and that could be one of the reasons why I've never been signed to a contract with any of the major porn production companies. I've never had time for all the petty politics and back-stabbing.

So here is the truth about how I got started in the glamorous profession that I'm in today, to the full

extent that I can actually understand it and make sense of it all myself!

The Spearmint Rhino guy who flew me from London lived in Houston, and after we touched down at the airport there he kindly put me up in a hotel for three nights. He even had his best friend, some pro-golfer guy, take me shopping, 'cause I had no clothes and no money! Then he flew me to Los Angeles with him and got me a separate room in the hotel where he was staying.

Within my first week of being in LA, he arranged my first gig – at a Spearmint Rhino, naturally enough. Unfortunately, it was in the worst possible location – the nowheresville of the City of Industry, in what Southern Californians call the Inland Empire. I hated it and didn't go back, because the guys there were sleazy and kept trying to grope me. There might not have been a six-foot rule like there was in London, but there was certainly a no-touching rule – it was just that some of the creeps in this place didn't know how to respect it.

After doing the gig, I had my benefactor drop me off at a hotel downtown – because I didn't realise that downtown was nowhere near Hollywood! And we said our goodbyes from there.

Fortunately, my agent in London had referred me to a really great photographer named Hank Londoner, and

I caught a cab to his studio in Culver City as soon as I could. When I got there, he told me he wanted to shoot me for adult magazines. And that's how my new career began, from London to Londoner! Hank was around 50 years old, with greyish long hair and a moustache and an interesting accent. (He had come to the United States from Israel and had started out in New York before moving to Los Angeles in 1997.) He was very well known for shooting for *Penthouse*, *Swank*, *Leg World* and many other magazines, and he had also started his own magazine, *New Rave*, in 1994.

Hank told me he wanted to photograph me exclusively, so I should get in touch with a guy called Roy Garcia. Roy would be my agent, and he would 'hold' me for after Hank got back from his upcoming two-week holiday. I found out that Roy Garcia had discovered a lot of major talent (Belladonna, Noname Jane, Bunny Luv and Kaylani Lei, to name just a few), so I thought 'what the hell' and rang him up. We arranged a meeting, and he came and met me outside my downtown hotel, as planned, and drove me to his place in Granada Hills. There, he asked me a deceptively simple question: 'Do you want to make a little money or a lot of money?'

I asked what a 'lot of money' would entail, and he said the magic word, 'Hardcore.'

I said, 'Sure, I'll try that.'

The single burning question most people want to ask a porn star is surely this: what were you thinking when you got into it?

Not everyone I meet actually asks it, but I'm sure they're thinking it. And the answer that a lot of the girls in the business will give you, if they're being honest, is 'I wasn't'. I know so, because I'm one of those girls.

Not a lot of deep thought went into it, at least not on any kind of conscious level. Saying I did it for the money or the drugs or the sex is only part of the answer. Those are really superficial reasons at best. Was I thinking? The truth is, I really had no goals coming into this industry. In the beginning, I did just do it for the money, and then it kind of grew on me. And I started to enjoy it, then I started to hate it, then enjoy it, then hate it, and I just keep going round and round with my emotions.

Another part of the answer is that porn was a great way for me to be able to become an actress, even if it wasn't the kind of acting I had intended on doing when I was growing up. But at least I got to live a part of my dream. And I also meant it as kind of a 'fuck you' to society and all the people who put me down. My new-found sense of glamour was sweet revenge on those who had ever made me feel like shit in the past.

When I made that critical decision to leave London and move so impulsively to Los Angeles, something was simmering in my brain. What I could never escape from was the fact that I had been teased my whole school life, until I was 14, about being skinny and poor and having big eyes. There were always people saying I would never amount to anything, because all I wanted to do was be a singer, dancer, actress and model. Even my own mother laughed and jeered at me. I guess this was my way of showing everyone what I was made of (quite literally, I guess!).

So here I was in LA, about to banish the ghosts of my abusive childhood and wipe the slate clean, post-London, post-Brisbane, post-everything from my first 20 years on the planet. I was going to start anew in Southern California and reinvent myself as Monica Mayhem.

It didn't take long for Roy to sign me up to shoot my first hardcore porn film, *Real Sex Magazine #38*. Bill Witrock was directing and I was starring opposite Lee Stone. Talk about in at the deep end! It was my very first time in more ways than one. I had never even seen a porn movie, I didn't know any names of any porn stars, and I didn't care. I do remember being a little self-conscious about whether or not I'd shaved properly! I didn't know how much pubic hair to leave in place, and I didn't even know about douching.

Roy explained to me what I needed to know about shooting porn. He was very professional about it, by which I mean there was no question of my having to have sex with him or anything. (And there were definitely no 'auditions', in case any of you were wondering!) At the time, I hadn't even had sex in front of a still camera – I hadn't done it with any kind of camera, still or moving, at all!

A few days later, Roy drove me to the set, which was at Bill's house, and I remember being so nervous. I had not had sex for almost a year, and he kept assuring me it would be easy. Bill was the cameraman as well as the director. He was nice and made me feel comfortable. I immediately received a vibe from him that he'd obviously done this a thousand times. 'Don't worry, Lee is a pro,' he said to me. 'He'll take good care of you. This is going to be really quick.'

I was led straight into make-up and was impressed at how glamorous the make-up artist made me look – much better and more natural than I'd looked in my softcore shoots in London.

Then in came Lee Stone – this huge, very buff and totally porno-looking guy who was very flirtatious, which made me feel comfortable and sexy. I had been worried at first, not knowing if I'd like the guy, but it turned out I was attracted to him, so everything was great! I actually don't remember much about the lead-up to the scene, but my jaw dropped when I saw him au naturel. His cock was so huge and it was very uniquely curved.

There were just three of us there in that room in Bill's house, and Lee and I did it on the bed. I had the guts to go through with it partly because it sounded so crazy – like, 'Wow, am I really doing this?' Lee was indeed a seasoned pro who knew what he was doing for the camera, so he pretty much just threw me into each position while Bill filmed and directed. It was over within an hour.

I can't remember much of it, other than my own feelings of being very unsure if I had done a good job or not. I knew full well how to have sex, of course, but I didn't know how to have sex for the camera. It was almost like being a virgin all over again. (Well, almost!)

I do remember peeing in the bathtub for some 'behind the scenes' footage. I thought that was a very odd thing to do and was a little uncomfortable doing it at first. But hey, I thought, I've peed in the bush many a time in front of friends, so what the hell!

So that was my first hardcore shoot. I got my cheque (for US$1500), and when Roy picked me up I told him I was ready to shoot more. I said to myself, and to Roy, 'If I don't like it, I'll stop doing it.'

It was that direct and straightforward for me. I know of strippers who say that they can take their clothes off and spread for men to see their pink but they'd never do porn. I'm the exact opposite. Spreading my thighs for a live audience is something I've done a lot, but I find it a little creepy sometimes. It's too up-close and personal, and I really have to get a little buzzed before going onstage and stripping to show my pussy. Porn is a lot more comfortable for me. I don't really think about the fact that guys are going to be watching the film and jerking off to me. The transition was pretty smooth, as far as I was concerned, and many people have said that I seemed more experienced than I actually was.

When Hank got back from his holidays, we shot some hardcore stills in his studio in Culver City, and I really enjoyed posing for him. They were long days but good days. I did some solo sets, some girl–girl and then boy–girl layouts. I was made up to look really glamorous, and again I remember thinking how unlike my tawdry modelling experiences in London this was. Everything was so amazingly professional – the make-up, the wardrobe and the sets – and I felt like a princess.

We did other sessions in other locations after that, and one in particular stands out. Hank took me and a male star named Nick Manning and some other chick (whose name I can't remember) to a gorgeous beach to shoot. We got stoned the whole time, and it was so much fun. A lot of sand found its way into everything – in places you don't want sand, if you get my drift – and the other girl, who was from England, kept complaining about it. I didn't take much notice of her. I was too busy fucking Nick Manning.

One of those photo sets was sold to *Australian Penthouse*, actually. It's crazy, but I never stopped to think that people who knew me back home – including, God forbid, my brother and father – could have seen those photos in Australia. I just wasn't in that sensible sort of headspace.

Because the turnover of new actors in these stills and movies is usually very, very high (the directors and photographers like fresh faces all the time), I thought I had to make the most of it while it lasted. In my first year, 2001, I found myself doing a lot of shoots – an average of 20 shoots a month – which meant that I had a *lot* of sex and certainly made up for lost time. I had no problem with throwing myself into it like this, but it took me at least six months to feel confident that I was actually giving a good performance.

A few bad reviews didn't help matters. Early on, a writer who was apparently not a fan of mine criticised me in every one of my scenes that he reviewed in *Adult Video News* (AVN), which is the main American adult-film-industry trade magazine. This really got to me. Back then, I would actually watch my movies and review my scenes to see what I could do better. And really, I couldn't see what was supposed to be so bad about them. I guess that guy had it in for me, or maybe he just wasn't a fan. Something like that can really hurt your career. It was only when I won a couple of awards and was getting loads of recognition that I started to feel more confident.

I won my first industry award in the same year that I'd started – the X-Rated Critics Organization (XRCO)

Award for 'Starlet of the Year' for 2001 – and then the Fans of X-Rated Entertainment (FOXE) 'Vixen of the Year' award in 2002. I was quite ambitious, actually, and I kept my mind on things like trying to get good reviews, good publicity, hot-looking box-covers, lots of magazine covers and, of course, making lots of money. Things like that kept me going, so I did feel very validated when I won. It was such an amazing affirmation, and I felt truly honoured and recognised for the hard work that I had put in.

But I was still so young and new to the business back then, and it didn't occur to me to think about whether there was some kind of disconnect between what the fans and critics felt about porn stars and what the girls themselves thought about the importance of such awards. I still don't really know, to be honest. To me, winning awards is just good publicity and recognition for a job well done, but I don't think the directors really give a shit. I came to this conclusion because I didn't get very much new work following those two awards. I don't think the real fans care, either, because those who really like you will like you regardless of whether you win awards or not.

That's not to say that I didn't do loads of work in 2002, though, because I was able to re-shoot for all the companies I'd already shot for, and for the same magazines, too. I hadn't hit the glass ceiling yet. I was still 'new' to lots of people.

But life wasn't always a bed of roses. I have my share of horror stories from my early days. There was one shoot in particular that was a nightmare. It was for a website, and I did it because it paid really well: US$350 an hour. It was really hard work and it took a bloody eternity. We shot it in Baltimore in one day, for about ten hours, and they wanted me to do all kinds of fucked-up shit, including using a speculum to allow the camera to get real 'tunnel vision'. They also shot me fucking myself with a bottle, followed by huge vegetables and sex toys. They thought I was just complaining but, seriously, I'm pretty tight down there and a fat butternut pumpkin is just not going to fit. I mean, how much more unnatural can a sex act be? I was trying to insert a big butternut pumpkin into my own vagina and pretending to enjoy it!

After I got back to LA, I was shooting for Hank Londoner again and I told a couple of girls there about the crazy things they made me do in Baltimore. They told this guy who'd shot me what I'd said, and he responded by threatening me in an email, calling me a cunt and saying he would sue me for slander, he would have me deported and this and that, blah, blah, blah. I had to smooth things over with a fake 'nice' email, explaining that I didn't badmouth him or his company but had only told those girls what I did there and it was entirely their own decision not to work with him after what they'd heard from me. That was a very weird experience.

In my early days in LA, my agent, Roy, had put me up at his house, where a bunch of other girls he represented lived. The first porn star I met there was Noname Jane, who was really sweet. She had a husband *and* a boyfriend, and I thought she was way cool. We're still good friends to this day. Jane is very spiritual and we have a lot in common. But most of the girls were complete crack-heads, straight out of Jerry Springer.

The girl I had to share a room with was a speed-smoking hooker. She was extremely stupid. She would walk Roy's two dogs in her stiletto heels at 2 am around Granada Hills, which is a genteel suburban area in the west San Fernando Valley, and she got her ID photo taken at the Department of Motor Vehicles wearing a stripper outfit, her head all cracked out. She was often offering guys blow jobs at the gym. She was just a filthy, messy pig who pretty much didn't sleep – a good thing, since I had to share a bed with her!

Another girl not only did speed and Ecstasy but was also the biggest pot smoker I'd ever seen. Her room was so disgusting – you couldn't even walk in there without stepping on something, including leftover food. Roy had to drive us to shoots and these girls were always one or two hours late. Naturally, Roy would blame all of us for this in front of the annoyed production managers at the shoots.

I was always professional, ready and waiting to go on time, but Roy was often so stressed out that he failed to give us the full story for a shoot, and this usually meant that we were unprepared. We went out not having the right clothes or we discovered that we weren't getting paid what we thought. And, to make things worse, Roy would often yell at people and fight and argue with his clients. Most people hated dealing with him. I lost a lot of work because many companies didn't want to book any girls through him.

The one ray of sunshine in my months living in Roy's house was meeting Belladonna, who was then calling herself just Bella. (She'd previously appeared in *Hustler* as 'Sandy' in 2000.) We got along instantly and started partying really hard. Roy wasn't getting us much work, so we had a lot of time on our hands. We would go out to clubs in Hollywood, get VIP treatment everywhere, go to after-parties – we totally ran amok.

Bella is originally from Utah and actually grew up a Mormon. She is two years younger than me and had been doing porn for about six months to a year before I'd got started. She had quit and moved back to Utah, then changed her mind and moved back to Roy's just after I'd moved there. I thought she was a very nice girl, and she went on to have an outstanding porn career. In 2003, at age 22, she decided to move on from acting to directing, for a well-known company called Evil Angel. Even back then, she already had quite a reputation for extreme sex, and she is known for putting huge objects up her ass and doing really hard, nasty scenes that often involve several guys gang-banging the bejeezus out of her. Of late, she has become somewhat notorious for slamming the industry on mainstream TV shows such as *20/20* and has been quite vocal about the health risks for its performers, having contracted chlamydia and gonorrhoea a few times herself. In 2005, she became a mother, with a healthy baby girl, and the baby shower was actually filmed and shown on *Family Business*, the Showtime reality series about the porn business.

But meantime, things began unravelling in the Roy Garcia house. One day, Roy came home from a trip and found we had stayed in and partied all night with the porn star Mark Davis. He lost it, as he'd specifically said that no parties and no guys were allowed in the house. I was trying to sleep and he kicked down the door, screaming at me. It was not a good scene, so Bella and I packed our bags and left. We stayed at the nearby Aku Aku Motel (21830 Ventura Boulevard, Woodland Hills, for those of you fans out there keen on tracing my chequered past).

With Roy out of the picture, we started representing ourselves. Bella was having a hard time getting work – somewhat hard to believe, given what an amazing performer she is, as everyone in porn now knows – so I was pumping her up to every director I was working for. Everyone was booking me for lead roles in features but no one liked Bella at the time because of her tattoos. I convinced a lot of people to hire her and we eventually moved in together to an apartment in Woodland Hills, got ourselves sober and started working hard.

A lot more work started coming in, which was great, even though I was often working up to 16 hours a day, five days a week. I scored an amazing role in a film for VCA Pictures called *The New Girl*. VCA told me that they hadn't used me before because they didn't want to deal with Roy as my agent. This film was directed by the great F. J. 'Freddie' Lincoln, who'd spent eight years directing for VCA until Larry Flynt took it over, and it was my first-ever lead role in a major feature film.

I loved this movie because it was set in the fourteenth century. I love period pieces, and in this one the costumes and settings were awesome. The storyline had my character drink a potion that put me to sleep for 400 years, and then I awoke in the basement of an internet voyeur-cam house, with porn stars all over the place. The best scene was when I snapped out of the fourteenth-century character and did two guys, Eric Price and Chris Cannon, and the hottest part of that threesome was when I was bouncing up and down in reverse-cowgirl position and giving a hot blow job at the same time.

It was about that time that I started dating a guy from Orange County, California, called Craven Moorehead (his stage name, obviously). The director Stoney Curtis had invited Bella and me to a club, and Craven was there because he was Stoney's production assistant at the time. We hit it off instantly. He was very sweet, though it wasn't until he invited me to a barbecue at Stoney's house in West Hills that I fell for him. We were alone, waiting for everyone else to show up, and he started playing my favourite song, Metallica's 'Fade to Black' from their *Ride the Lightning* album. I mean, he was playing it perfectly on guitar, because it was his favourite song too.

And then, by sheer chance, Metallica's *Garage Days Re-Revisited* EP came on the radio! That did it. The song 'Last Caress/Green Hell', written by Glenn Danzig, just slays me, and the whole thing ends with those Iron Maiden riffs (actually, it's Metallica's parody of Iron Maiden's 'Run to the Hills'). Iron Maiden was another of my favourite bands when I was growing up. Juvenile-delinquent headbanger heaven. Craven and I just connected immediately!

Bella, however, didn't like Craven and me being together at all; she knew what a player he was. Everyone in the industry knew about him, because he was always hitting on girls. Bella had seen him out with other girls when we were dating, too, so his reputation as a horndog was always out there for all to see. I guess I knew, intuitively, that Bella was right, but I truly hoped he could change.

While personally things were tricky, my career was going from strength to strength, and I was getting more great roles. In 2002, I starred in *Perfect*, directed by Michael Ninn for Private Media Group, which was described as a '*Matrix*-style hardcore blockbuster packed with high-tech special effects' in Private's 2002 mail-order catalogue.

I played a robot, since it was a very futuristic movie, and I had some crazy hair and make-up done by one of my favourite make-up artists, Lee Garland. I wore a very sexy white, full-body leotard and did some robot-like dialogue in a dream-like state with smoke all around, and then did a scene with Dale DaBone on a steel table. We had some crazy sex against a green screen while suspended in the air with harnesses. It was supposed to look like *The Matrix*, as I'm leaning back in mid-air, getting fucked. (It was a lot of fun on the harness and I would have loved to have done all kinds of tricks!)

At the end of the shoot, it was very stressful for the crew and for Dale because Michael had this crazy idea about how to shoot the pop shot – he lined up 20 cameras in a circle around us and they were all supposed to go off simultaneously and continuously while Dale was cumming. It was supposed to look like slow motion all around, and it resulted in one of the longest sex scenes I've ever shot. I'm not sure if it came out the way that Michael had it planned but it was certainly a very unique way of ending a sex scene. What a climax!

Somehow, during this hectic period of my life, Craven and I found ourselves driving to Las Vegas to get married. Bella and Craven's best friend, Dez, were in the car with us, and they were going to be our bridesmaid and best man. Craven was at the wheel and I was sitting behind – we'd had a big fight just before we left, and he'd refused to let me, his future bride, sit next to him in the car en route to our wedding! (Hmm. Was that an omen or what?)

Let me say now, with the wisdom of hindsight, that I think getting married on a whim is a bit insane, to say the least. (I don't recall being on drugs at that point, but I did start up again after I got married.) As strange as it may sound, we had made the decision a whole two weeks before heading out to Vegas. I remember thinking to myself, 'Is this really a good idea?' But then I decided to do it anyway, thinking what harm could it do. (I could always get a divorce if things didn't work out, right?) So we got married at the Viva Las Vegas wedding chapel, which I had pre-booked. I rented a beautiful dress, and Craven rented a tuxedo. And Bella looked ravishing as my bridesmaid, as she always did.

When we got back to LA after the wedding, I was still living with Bella, as Craven and I hadn't yet found a place together. But Bella then let another porn star move in with us and that completely fucked up my whole friendship with her. This girl (who will remain nameless) was obsessed with Bella and she was jealous of me and my career. She would monopolise Bella's time, and they excluded me to do their own thing together, often walking out and slamming the door without even saying goodbye. In the end, I couldn't stand it any more, and it was a great relief when I moved in with Craven. Bella and I never made up after that whole incident, which is a real shame because she was such a good friend.

And so began my period of domestic bliss with Craven. Ha! To cut a woefully long story mercifully short, my marriage was a two-and-a-half year disaster. It led to me nearly ruining my career during what was to have been my peak time, shortly after I got my boobs enlarged in 2002. And I would much rather talk about my boobs than talk about my ex-husband, so I hope you will bear with me here.

Ever since I'd stopped growing at 16, I had wanted bigger breasts. So in LA, as soon as I finally had plenty of money to spend, I asked around and talked to a few girls in the business who had nice boobs. Among the famous porn stars, Jill Kelly had my favourite set of boobs, so I decided to go to her surgeon, Dr Fischer (who is now on the TV show *Extreme Makeover*). I was able to afford being out of work for a couple of months, so I stayed completely sober for the first month, got my boobs done and continued staying sober during the month-long recovery period. (Then I made up for lost time and partied hard on New Year's Eve!)

Looking back, I can say it was the scariest, most painful experience I've ever had. It was scary being put under anaesthesia, and it was painful from the minute

I woke up. All I remember is coming out of surgery, hearing the nurses but not being able to see them yet, and then figuring out that what they were saying was, 'Stop kicking, you'll cause bleeding!' I was kicking around, trying to wake up. Then I opened my eyes and said, 'Is it done yet?' Apparently, I didn't notice the huge mountain on my chest, not until the pain kicked in and I had to have more morphine, which knocked me out again. The swelling takes a long time to go down, and then your boobs don't really drop for about a year – that's when they start looking more natural. And, as the years go by, your boobs tend to look smaller than they first appeared, but I'm very proud of them now. That was my one and only boob job.

My bigger chest immediately made me feel way more confident with myself, and I really had a great time going shopping for a change. It felt so awesome to walk into Victoria's Secret knowing I was able to buy a D-cup bra! And I could pretty much wear any kind of top, whereas when I had small boobs I had the worst time trying to find tops that made me feel sexy. Now I felt like more of a woman.

Armed with my new self-confidence, I started feature-dancing that year, and I eventually got more gigs than I could handle. I made a ton of money. Feature-dancing is when a stripper gets paid per show to be the headline act at a gentlemen's club. Usually, this girl is a porn star, and her name and celebrity will draw more customers to the club. A feature dancer will always put on a much more elaborate show than a regular dancer – with big, expensive costumes, props, games, merchandise and other stuff. I was dancing my ass off in the strip clubs across the country.

In all fairness, Craven can't take full responsibility for the problems in my movie career. It's true that I worked condom-only after we were married, and I lost a lot of work because of it – people don't want to shoot condoms. We did have some kind of co-dependence thing going on, though, which was sometimes indirectly detrimental to me. There were a couple of times, for instance, when Craven didn't like who I was working with – meaning, he didn't like me fucking certain guys – so I acquiesced and didn't do those shoots. He once insisted that I come out to some stupid car show with him, so I had to cancel work. Then, there was our constant fighting, which sometimes led me to cancel shoots too.

When I was going through all of this emotional turbulence, I would sometimes turn to cocaine to numb the pain. I wanted to kick the habit, though, and I went through a stage when I would have it in my possession for months at a time and not even touch it. I thought I had it under control, but I was just about to enter another period of partying.

Marriage, clearly, wasn't quite the panacea I had hoped for. Eventually, in December 2003, we split up and Craven moved out. It wasn't all doom and gloom, because it had been on the cards for ages, and a room in my house that I'd been renting out became vacant not too long after, and Jay Allan, my good friend and favourite photographer, moved in. Let the good times roll! Boy, we had some great house parties.

Chapter Five

CALIFORNICATION

People have asked me what I think, in retrospect, is the most important lesson I learned about making the transition from modelling to movies. Sometimes, I'm not sure how to answer that. The thing is, I do love modelling and I wish I could have done more mainstream magazine layouts, such as *Maxim* or *FHM*.

Actually, if I hadn't done hardcore, I could have tried out for *Playboy* magazine, which would have probably launched a whole different career for me. Perhaps it would have led me to mainstream acting and modelling, which is what I really wanted. But *Playboy* likes to deploy its famous 'girl next door' branding, and usually doesn't use us 'girls gone bad' hardcore models. This helps to distinguish it from its main competitor, *Penthouse*, which uses adult film stars a great deal in pictorials and centrefolds (and which I've appeared in loads). The one time *Playboy* made a notable exception was in its March 2002 issue, when they did a cover story and pictorial on 'The Women of Porn' and they had three Vivid Video contract girls (Tera Patrick, Kira Kener and Dasha) on the cover. Things could have been different, I guess, but being a Pisces I'm often too hasty with my decisions, and that's always been my biggest problem. In so many ways, I am my own worst enemy.

That's not to say that I'm not grateful for how quickly I was able to make an impact on the porn industry. This might have been because I was one of the few Australian girls shooting porn in the US, a market where very few non-American girls were being employed. There were the Aussies Jodie Moore and Bobbi Barrington, too, but they were only just coming into the industry around the same time as me.

The path I took was to base myself in Southern California and work my ass off, whereas Jodie wanted to be the number-one Aussie porn star so bad that she ran for a seat in the Queensland parliament in 2001 and the Australian senate in 2004 – which, if you ask me, is an easy way to get famous. She can't have realistically believed that she'd be voted in. From what I've witnessed, when girls in our industry do these kinds of things, it's seen by most people as a publicity stunt. As a result, people lose respect for girls like us. But Jodie was clearly of another school of thought – any publicity is good publicity, right? And as for Bobbi Barrington, she made a small splash doing 'gonzo' porn and did well for a while, although she seems to have vanished from the scene almost as quickly as she came in. I have no idea where she is today.

Gonzo, by the way, is a sub-genre of hardcore porn that's half-improvised theatre, half-reality TV, whereby performers work without a script and have to make stuff up as they go along, including the sex, which often doesn't have a director calling fixed positions. Usually, it is shot cheaply with a very small crew, often a single cameraman with a hand-held camera. The resulting 'amateur' effect is part of its appeal, as is the 'shock value' of performers having spontaneous sex with real people suddenly roped into scenes. The creation of gonzo porn is often credited to the famous director John Stagliano.

Bobbi did a scene in a 2001 VCA Pictures production in which I had the leading role, *Portrait of a Woman*. Bobbi's appeal was obvious, since she was a big-breasted blonde who totally fit the preferred porn-star stereotype. We once did a photo shoot together for the photographer Suze Randall, in which I dominated her. I was dressed up as a 1940s Mafia chick. It was a smokin' hot layout, but I'm not sure where it ended up. I would have loved to have seen that magazine. We don't always know where our shoots end up, unless we want to spend time at news-stands looking at porno magazines, hoping to see ourselves on the cover! I don't do that, of course, and usually find out which magazines I'm in through my fans telling me.

As I've said, posing for magazines was one of my favourite things to do at first. I particularly loved posing for Suze Randall, for whom I probably did at least 20 layouts. Suze is hysterical. She's British, a great photographer and was originally a *Playboy* model. She was always really loud during photo shoots. She would say funny things like, 'Spread your legs, you lazy sheila!' or, 'Point your toes, bitch!' It was (and still is) rare to have a female photographer shoot you in this business. The other female photographer whom I really liked is Robbye Bentley. She is a really crazy character too. Robbye did a lot of my early shoots in 2000 and 2001 (before moving into directing porn films, as you've seen at the start of this book). I loved posing for her.

Among the female movie directors, I really like Kelly Holland. Kelly is just really cool and laid-back. She's very easy to work with, knows what she wants and gets great results. I remember having her as a cinematographer during the shoots I did with VCA, and then eventually she became a director. She hails from Dallas, Texas, and was at first a mainstream actress with a trained theatrical background and then became a mainstream documentary director before she moved to shooting porn. (She has actually done serious documentaries, for her company Art Attack Productions, on a variety of fascinating subjects, including two she shot in Latin America about military coups and the fanaticism of soccer fans – a whole world away from porn!) Kelly got the break of her career when Vivid Video hired her to direct movies, which she did for seven years under the name Toni English. She then directed for another big porn company, Adam & Eve, under the same name before working under her real name in 2004 at Playgirl. ('I started directing under my name with Playgirl because I couldn't tell women to "claim their sexuality" and then work under a pseudonym,' she said.) She moved to Penthouse in 2005 and became its head of production before assuming her current position as president of Penthouse Studios.

I like both Kelly and Suze not because they're women who are successful in what has always been a male-dominated business but because they're both very good at what they do, period. I see no reason why a woman can't deliver the goods from behind the camera as well as any man.

As far as other porn stars go, I've always thought Shayla LaVeaux was awesome, and the way she is still performing for the camera after the age of 35 is inspiring. I love Shayla's attitude, since she's so friendly and down to earth and never seems to let anything get to her head. But as a whole, I can truthfully say that no one inspired me to get into the business. I didn't know any names before coming in. Afterwards, I watched some of Jill Kelly's scenes and got to know her, and she gave me some good advice – including the breast-surgeon tip-off – which helped me a lot. In some ways, I wanted to be like Jill. I just thought she was so hot! When she walked into a room, you could feel her sexy energy. I learned from Jill that sexual energy is contagious.

In an interview I gave in 2006 to *Eve*, a mainstream women's magazine in London, I said that the most important technique that all aspiring porn stars need to learn is 'to open your legs so the camera can see the sex'. It's actually a lot harder than it seems. It's more than spreading your own lips with your hand. It means opening up your angle to the camera when you're having sex so the viewers can see the 'hardcore' at all times – knowing how to keep your thighs spread no matter what position you're holding, so that the camera can see the guy's penis penetrating you (if that's what's going on). To do this, you have to be constantly aware of where the camera is in relation to the heart of the action – and nobody ever has to consider this when they're having sex at home!

In porn, you have to learn to expose your body in ways most women would be too shy to actually do but which, if they're honest with themselves, they might well fantasise about. I think we do fulfil a vicarious need for women who enjoy watching our movies. So, over the first couple of years in the business, I developed a professional skill set, in the same way that Maria Sharapova works on her serve and her backhand. I eventually just got used to these new ways of having sex, and I became more flexible after doing it for a while, especially from so many photo shoots where I needed to hold the positions. I well and truly lost my porn virginity.

Doing reverse-cowgirl, for example, is a great leg workout and fantastic for cardio. It's a porn position where the guy lies down flat on his back and the girl gets on top but facing away from him. This is considered a good camera shot for obvious reasons: she's facing the camera with her legs spread apart, so viewers can see the total full-frontal exposure, what we call the 'insertion shot', of his erect penis going in and out of her open vagina.

Yoga really helps, too: it tones the body and makes you look good. I have no problem spreading for the camera these days. It just happens naturally, because I instinctively know I have to open up for the light. If I see darkness down there, I find the light – pretty crazy, huh?

I'm sure there are women who must think I'm a lunatic, because there's just no way in hell they could ever imagine themselves doing what I do for a living. I can understand them not wanting people to watch them have sex, but I guess that's where the actress side of me comes into play. You really do have to be a good actress. At first, I felt very uncomfortable with the idea of people watching, but then I thought, 'Wait, I'm an actress. I'm not just having sex in front of the camera, I'm performing!' So I think about my performance and how I'm reacting, and it's always great when you actually enjoy working with someone. You kind of get lost in that moment and forget about everyone around you, until the director yells out 'Cut!' or 'Next position!' – usually just as you're about to cum for real. I hate it when that happens!

The other thing that's hard to explain to anyone who hasn't worked in this industry is how demanding it can be physically and how it can affect your domestic life. When I was married to Craven and shooting a lot, I was always sore and I didn't want to have sex off-camera, because I didn't want to be in pain shooting the next day. So the balance was tough. It was a good thing he loved blow jobs!

The thing about our relationship was that Craven was primarily not a performer but a camera guy, someone who shot stuff and was graduating to directing gonzo porn. Craven already had his own blow-job series, called *The Oral Adventures of Craven Moorehead*, and he had appeared in a couple of scenes elsewhere in the past. By the time he got round to directing me, our relationship was pretty dead anyway, so I didn't much care about fucking someone in front of him. We did perform one blow-job scene together and a sex scene with another girl, so I can't say that counts as jointly performing all that much. Really, it was just another job to both of us.

One of my favourite films from my early years of porn was *Sweet Sounds*, directed by Nicholas Steele. I was the lead in this 2003 movie, which received several five-star reviews. It was about a singer trying to get her big break, and the song they had me sing in it was a ballad, which they wouldn't let me sing the way I wanted to but it ended up sounding great anyway. I did three hot sex scenes and a lot of actual acting, and the most notable scene features me and Cheyne Collins on a rooftop in downtown LA at night, in the middle of winter – it was freezing and we were exhausted by the time we had to have sex, but it looked so hot. I always loved shooting with Cheyne – he's good-looking, very cool and easy to work with. (And he has a perfect cock – not too big, and not too small. Give me the average-sized ones any time!*)

That same year, 2003, I got my first writing credit on a movie, which was a huge deal for me. The movie was *Witch Coven College* and it was directed by the late, great Jim Holliday for VCA. It was basically a spoof about witches teaching college girls a few tricks, although it was pure fantasy and nothing truly of a Wiccan nature. But it was so much fun to shoot. We had 'magic dust' that

---

* By average here, I mean average for porn, not for normal life, as in around six to eight inches.

made people automatically have sex, so it was intended as comedy, just like all of Jim's movies. There were a lot of hot chicks, a lot of toe-sucking, butt-licking, anal and girl–girl scenes. I wrote the script around Jim's sense of humour, and he loved it. Of course, he would add his own words and phrases, which he always enjoyed doing. I still think of this movie as my way of paying homage to him.

Jim was such a treasure and we worked together for several years, until he died in December 2004. He used to call me one of his 'angels', which is a term of endearment that he used for the top girls who appeared in his movies. Among those top girls were Jill Kelly, Shayla LaVeaux and Felecia, so of course I was honoured to be included in that company. Eventually, he started to call me his number-one angel (replacing my idol Jill Kelly), and as I was the only one of his angels who didn't do anal that was a great honour for me.

Jim always liked to put me in the middle of the box-covers and almost always had me as the lead girl. And when I decided I was quitting the business, right at the peak of my career, Jim would pay me just to walk around in one of his movies and have me show off my butt!

Working for Jim was a great experience. There were always 15 to 20 girls on set, and Jim had his quirky way of shooting things. I'll always remember that he loved pink lipstick and pink nail polish, and he would have us wear moccasins sometimes, as part of his trademark.

In 2003, he directed another of my screenplays, *Charm School Brats*. Both *Charm School Brats* and *Witch Coven College* got great reviews and turned out really cool.

It was very sad when Jim died. Jim had diabetes, but the catering was never very healthy on his sets. It was 'Jimmyland', as he called it, and what Jimmy wanted Jimmy got. He always said he'd be surprised if he lived to be 50, but he made it to 55. Hustler eventually took over VCA, and things changed. I was no longer shooting big features for them and they were thinking of cutting Jim's movies out all together, which shocked me because they were apparently the best-selling movies that VCA had to offer.

The porn-star work kept coming in during this time, but I couldn't quite hit my stride again in terms of reviews and notices, almost as if I'd peaked and had to hit the brakes before I crashed. I freaked out at that juncture and took a hiatus. There was a lull in 2003 when I worked less and less, and I didn't resurrect myself until 2004.

Absolute Mayhem

Abducted by aliens but still masturbating! In Darren Kaye's *Hysteria*, 2001.

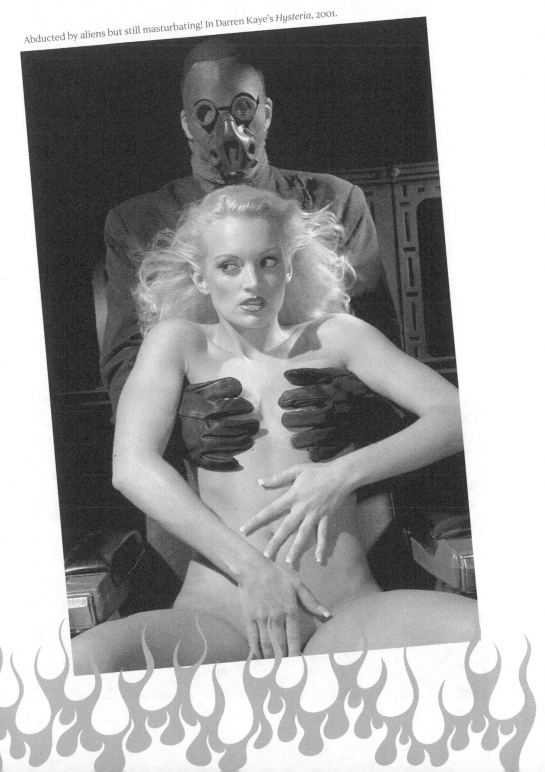

Monica Mayhem

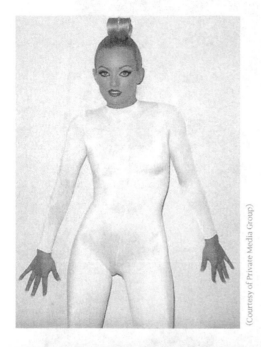

Yours truly, the pure-white robot.
In Michael Ninn's *Perfect*, 2002.

Sleeping beauty (for 400 years),
in my first big feature, F. J. Lincoln's
The New Girl, 2001.

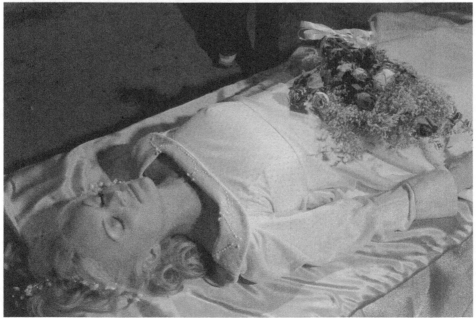

(Top) Lubin' my vibe before use and lovin' it! On the set of *Skin*, 2003.

(Bottom) Black is the new black! With director John Strong on the set of *Rain Coater's Point of View #9*, 2008.

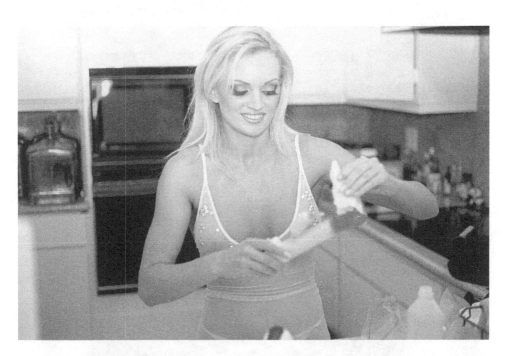

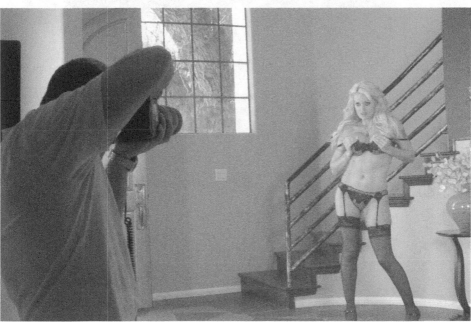

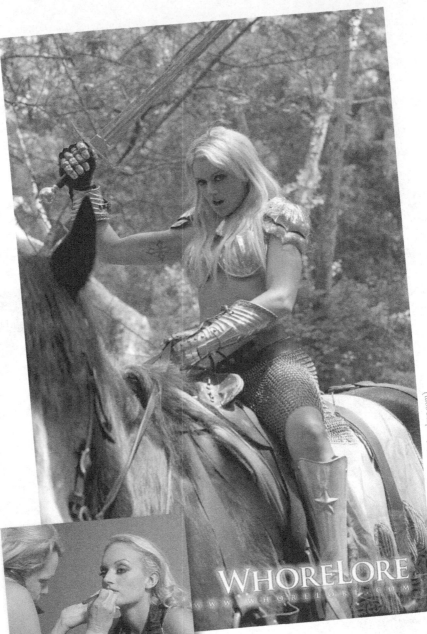

Reliving my medieval past life. On the set of *Whorelore*, 2008.

The only time I can ever sit still, in make-up! On the set of *Amber's Pursuit*, 2002.

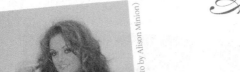

(photo by Alison Minion)

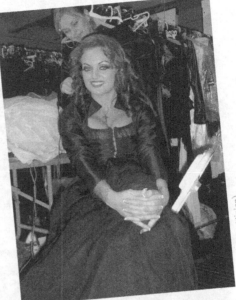

(photo by Alison Minion)

Hair done, script read, waiting to
go to work! On *Sacred Sin*, 2006.

All gussied up and finally kitted out!
On *Sacred Sin*, 2006.

'Uh, you want me to do *what* with the
boom mic?' On *Haven's Magic Touch 2*,
with director Bud Lee (left) and actor
T. J. Cummings (middle), 2001.

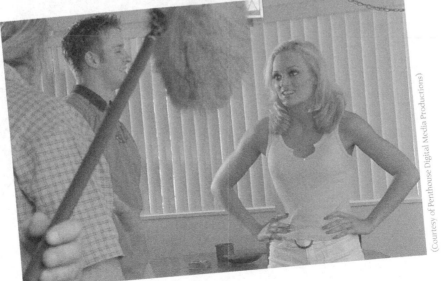

(Courtesy of Penthouse Digital Media Productions)

Who needs *Twilight*? As a vampire dominatrix in *Dark Angels 2: Bloodline*, 2005.

(Photo by Red Ezra)

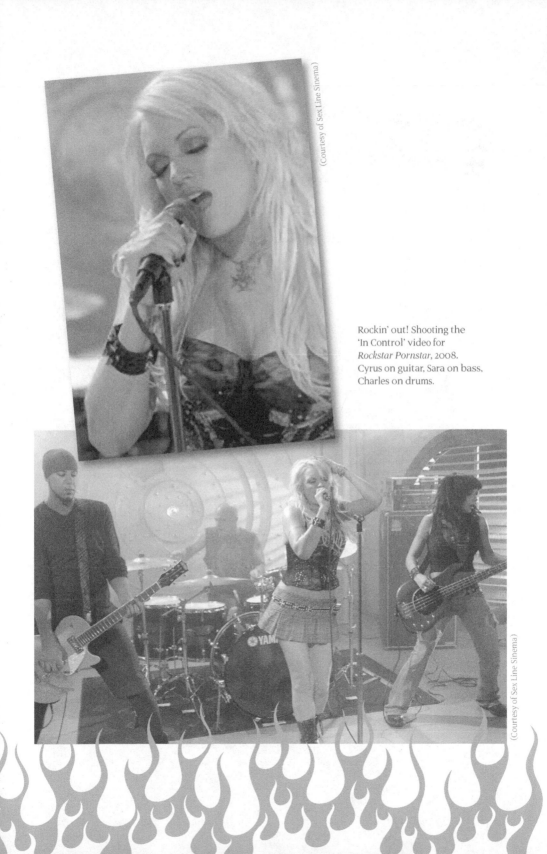

Rockin' out! Shooting the 'In Control' video for *Rockstar Pornstar*, 2008. Cyrus on guitar, Sara on bass, Charles on drums.

And I do like 'em rock hard! The DVD box-cover for *Rockstar Pornstar*, 2008.

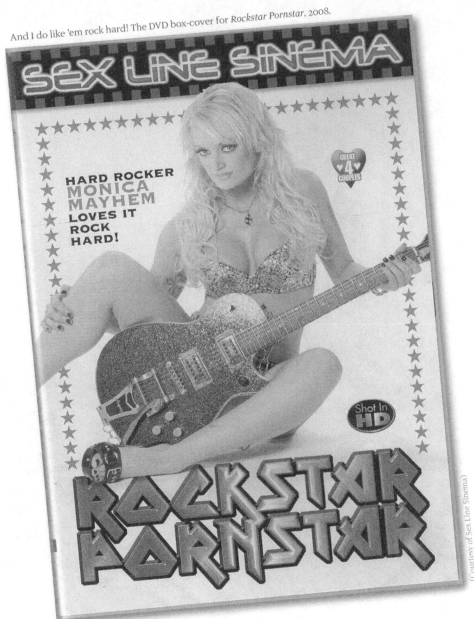

Chapter Six

MAINTAINING
CONTROL

*A*fter four years as a porn star, I had achieved such fame as an adult-film actress that it had translated into increased demand for me as a feature dancer. That's how it works: success as a porn star is what gets you the feature billing at a strip club, and that can be very lucrative. I was dancing in clubs across the USA and Canada and was also flown out to Melbourne, to dance at the Spearmint Rhino there, where I shook my booty to the music of Australian bands such as AC/DC and INXS. (As a feature dancer, you do get to choose your own music.) My dance career became hugely successful, and for a long time it was my biggest source of income.

I've got some great stories about my experiences on the dance stage. You know that famous phrase from NASA, 'Houston, we have a problem'? Well, one time I was featuring in Houston, Texas, and while I was on stage I suddenly noticed some guy jacking off, right at the tip rail! I laughed and pointed him out to the bouncers, who began freaking out. They started discussing among themselves who was going to go up to the guy to tell him to stop. One of them eventually went up and said, 'Listen, sir, you can't do that in here. You're going to have to leave.' I mean, he had his cock out in public, right there, by my tip rail – I thought it was so fucking hilarious but also gross at the same time!

That was the only time this happened to me, but there have been other kinds of dance-stage drama. I've had bouncers run up to grab guys who have jumped up on stage, and I've also had to slap guys for grabbing me. One guy even bit my nipple, and I responded by hitting him really hard. (Most women defend themselves against sexual harassment at work, but my methods take that to a whole new level!)

At its peak, the porn-star life involves balancing life on the road with filming. I actually loved mixing shooting and dancing – that way I wouldn't get bored with one or the other. But there are things you need to do in order to cope with that lifestyle.

One night in 2007, at The Crazy Horse in San Francisco, I nearly collapsed before my first show.

I'm sure it was due to my unhealthy, stressful lifestyle: drinking, lack of sleep and not eating right are a bad combination. And the random panic attacks I'd been having weren't helping either, not to mention almost having an asthma attack from all the strippers chain-smoking backstage. But I still went on stage that night, a little late. I finished up three very low-energy shows still feeling dizzy. I was actually scared I might fall over and pass out.

After the show, I met the cutest 18-year-old who had seen all my movies and wanted to get into porn. I told her to finish school and call me before she did anything in this business. I could have easily made a ton of money off her by setting myself up as her agent, but something came over me. I didn't want to be the person responsible for potentially ruining this girl's life. A lot of girls might be emotionally stable enough to handle this industry, but some girls end up wrecking their lives with drugs. Instead, I gave her advice on how not to go off the rails while being a porn star and on the consequences that she would suffer for the rest of her life. I've learned so much from my years of experience yet I'm still picking up the pieces of my life. I hope that girl listened to me. I know there are a lot of directors who will be pissed off when they hear that. But I really don't care what anyone thinks. I was doing a good deed, giving some good advice, something for her to think about before she jumps into this world.

I find it very flattering when new girls come up to me all star-struck, and I'm always willing to give them advice so they don't make some of the same mistakes I did – like partying all your money away and helping out people who turn out to be less than true friends. Basically, I tell them just to be wary of everyone and not to do anything that they're not comfortable with. Maintaining control of your career is the key.

I hate seeing these girls that come in and do scenes for practically nothing. We deserve way more than what we get paid, and some of the new girls who work for low rates just spoil it for everyone. And the girls who come in and say, 'I wanna be the next Jenna,' they really make me laugh. They are so naive. Those days are long gone. Jenna Jameson was a publicity machine. She came into the business at the right time and had the right people behind her, back when there weren't nearly as many girls in the industry as there are today. These little girls can't seem to grasp that fact.

The truth, though, is that they do have youth and time on their side. Agents today like to offer producers new girls to shoot, because new girls pay a higher percentage in the beginning and the agents win on commission. I miss the days when there weren't so many agents and I'd constantly get calls for work from production managers.

From 2002 to 2005, although I was at the top of my game professionally – successfully combining dancing and filming – it was hard because I could never book a shoot within a few days of coming back into town. My body was always too beaten up from dancing, and I felt so bruised and sore. I needed to relax and get massages and heal myself. It's part of the whole process of taking care of business.

I was also doing a lot of partying, which for me involved consuming too much alcohol, cocaine, marijuana and Xanax. Deep down, I was just sick of porn in general: I had worked too much too soon. It was all starting to become a blur and I found that depressing. I realised I was going through an early mid-life crisis of sorts, just three years short of turning 30.

I was also starting to think that I might have chosen the wrong profession – I wanted to be a rock star, not a porn star, and it finally occurred to me that I may have ruined that ambition for myself. So I tried to sabotage my porn career by being rebellious. I had the dragon from the Welsh national flag tattooed on my upper left arm, as my way of saying '*Cymru am byth!*' ('Wales forever!') and '*Y Ddraig Goch ddyry cychwyn!*' ('The red dragon will show the way!'), as all good Welshpersons are wont to proclaim. I had lost touch with my heritage over the years, and as I have always strongly identified with my Welsh ancestry it was a great way of getting back in touch with who I really was. Except, of course, a lot of porn producers don't like tattoos and wouldn't hire me. What's more, I was known in the porn world as a blonde, but I went and became a redhead, to make me look more like a rock star. And all that did was create problems for my public image.

People didn't want to shoot me as a redhead with tattoos because they thought the fans would either not recognise me or, worse, hate me for my new look. It was a complete mistake on my part and I admit I really fucked up. I still hadn't learned that there's a difference between your public persona and your personal self, and if you want to be a celebrity of any sort you have to somehow manage to keep both in check.

Yet you can only go so far. There are cases in which your private self and public persona do have to be in harmony, otherwise you risk losing sight of your identity. For instance, I've done a fair number of scenes involving sexual fetishes and also bondage and domination. In real life, I don't like to dominate guys, because I want them to take charge, to act like a real man. But I do love to dominate women. After all, I am a bit of a tomboy at heart.

I've worked for Cybernet in San Francisco a couple of times – a company that runs lots of bondage websites – and for one of the scenes I had to beat the crap out of a girl. She was the porn star Ariel X, and she loves that kind of thing. (Each to their own, I guess.) Then I got sent on a shoot for a fetish site, Fetishnation.com. My agent told me that it would only be some light bondage and spanking, so I accepted. When I got to the set, they explained everything they were going to do to me – they would tie me down and then force me to orgasm while slapping and whipping me and pulling my hair, as well as verbally humiliating me. I totally freaked out. I told them I couldn't be submissive. I was afraid it would stir up some old feelings from the past – of being abused, mentally and physically. They were very nice people and said they didn't want me to do it if I was at all uncomfortable, though they were understandably pissed at my agent for sending someone who 'doesn't do submissive'! So that was one instance where the public persona and the private self had to mesh perfectly or it just wasn't going to work.

I do love getting dressed up for fetish shoots, though, especially if I'm going to be wearing latex, which looks all shiny but grips your skin at the same time. I wore a slinky black latex number for a Penthouse movie called *Fetish Diaries*, released in April 2007. It featured me doing light bondage stuff with a male slave, played by the porn star Van Damage. I remember that it was very hot – it must've been 38°C in that studio – and I was dripping with sweat. It would just pour out of me every time I took a piece of latex clothing off, and I had to gradually undress to complete the scene, which involved me sucking and fucking the slave.

I also did some bizarre fetish stuff for Taylor St Claire, who not only is one of the best porn stars in the business but also has a second career as a professional *domme*.

I've always thought her such a sexy woman, all natural and curvy, and she looks so beautiful, like a soap-opera star or something. One of her scenes involved me teasing a submissive male slave, who had the smallest penis I've *ever* seen. In real life, he's actually Taylor's slave and he's into that kind of thing for real – he was telling me what kind of mean things I should say to him, and I felt so bad. I mean, his penis was tiny and I had to point and laugh at it and make him feel like shit.

Then I shot some scenes for this sneezing-fetish website that Taylor had called *Sneezing Beauties*. I had to tickle my nose with a toothpick until I sneezed five times. And then I was filmed blowing my nose. I can't believe there is actually a fetish for that. But there really are guys out there who will get off on seeing me sneeze and blow my nose, and they will actually pay the current rate – seven bucks for a five-minute, 38-megabyte wmv file – to see me do so. They'll get all excited and masturbate at the sight of my nasal mucus. Good heavens, if they knew I was really asthmatic some of them might orgasm right away!

Another time, I did a photo shoot where I was bound and put in a coffin filled with nails. That was kind of creepy. And the coffin was suspended too. I couldn't move and had no control over anything. I freaked out a little, because I hate not being in control.

And control is something that is getting harder and harder to keep hold of in the world of porn. These days, the rates are getting lower and lower because the industry has been undergoing an awful recession in these past few years, and that means porn stars are less able to pick and choose which jobs they feel comfortable about taking.

The explosion of gonzo porn that occurred right after I started out, back in 2001, has been largely responsible for this downturn. Call me old-fashioned, but I'm still a believer in movies as art, and today we live in an age where our art form has been desecrated in the name of greed. The year I got into the business marked the end of the big-features era, and gonzo was starting to make its way into the rental market in a very big way. The onslaught of gonzo is what has killed the industry. Too many companies got greedy because they thought it was easy – because gonzo is unscripted 'reality' porn that is cheap to shoot – but they didn't realise how many other companies were getting into the game too, and thus everyone ended up fighting for their slice of the same pie. A lot of companies went bust in the summer of 2007 and some are barely alive at this point.

People downloading free porn off the internet is the other sure thing that's killing our industry. It's bad enough that we porn stars don't get paid nearly enough for what we're worth, what with all the health-and-safety risks we take, but now we're getting paid even less – because the companies are making less money from their products. That's the grim reality from where

I sit on my career-transitioning perch, as we roll into 2009 and observe the market meltdown happening all over the world. (My heart sank at the end of 2008 as I watched the Australian dollar plunge to its lowest value in years!)

Ironically, this doesn't seem to have stemmed the massive flow of new girls coming into the business. In the past year, I have gone to sets and read entire call sheets where I don't even recognise a single name. These new girls seem to arrive by the truckload from Tennessee to Texas, and it often stuns me to realise that I have to compete with them for places in movies.

We're all forced to work for less money as the film-production pile continues to shrink, so where is this industry really heading? When I started out, I got paid US$1400 for an oral-orgy scene (a blow-bang, as it's known in the trade), which is actually a little more than the usual rate (though it's nowhere near enough, given what's involved). At this time of writing, I'm getting paid US$400 for a regular blow job, doing just one guy, though it used to be US$500 when the economy was better. A lot of girls in the business will now blow guys on film for only US$300 or less.

Lack of control of our image is another issue we porn stars face. One good example is when they use bad pictures of me. There have been so many box-covers on which I think I look hideous. I just don't understand what's wrong with the people who chose those pictures. I know for a fact that there are always some beautiful photos of me in every set that's shot, and yet someone with one eye gets to choose the worst of the bunch for public display – like the ones where they show me putting a huge cock in my mouth on the cover, with my cheek all stretched out. Most consumers make impulse decisions based on what they see, and it's really important for my branding to get my look right. However, the reality of this business is that you're at the mercy of the art department at the studio, and there's a train of thought that the nastiest shots are the best. It's just that sometimes these people forget about the girl who's at the receiving end of what's being shot.

Another example of this lack of control of my image was the occasion I did an internet-TV show, in which I was filmed blowing Dez, who had become one of my best friends despite having been best man at my ill-fated wedding to Craven. I didn't really want to do it, because I had to go out right after that and I didn't want to have to re-do my make-up. So it was a held-back kind of blow job, and when he was about to cum I opened my mouth really wide so that he would get it in there and not on my face. I kept my mouth open for about ten seconds, right until he came, and then he did it on my boobs instead. Anyway, they took a still of the mouth-open-wide shot and they kept showing it throughout the show, on high-rotation, like it was supposed to be funny.

I didn't think it was funny at all. I thought I looked terrible, and not exactly the epitome of grace and beauty, to be sure. I don't think that's cool at all. I have to look good and hot for the fans: they can't be showing me looking like some stupid, slobbering, sex-starved whore.

But you also have to keep a sense of humour about yourself, in order to maintain your sanity in this business. Someone recently showed me the box-cover for one of my old movies, *Uninhibited*, directed by F. J. Lincoln, which this person had acquired in London. This was the British VHS-version box-cover, made by Hot Rod Productions, which was startlingly different from the American version. They'd used old photos of me from an earlier era of my career, taken from a different movie altogether, when my hair was bright blonde and straight, rather glamorous-looking, and juxtaposed them with a main photo of my co-star Evan Stone sticking his middle finger into my exposed vagina, which was completely shaved for the viewer's maximum ogling pleasure. There are two smaller inset photos of penises jammed into vaginas (not mine) and the spine of the box had a shot from the movie of me with my tongue lovingly lapping a very erect cock (belonging to Marty Romano, who did the opening scene with me).

What can you do, you know?

These companies will do their utmost to sell a movie the best way they can, appealing to the baser instincts of the potential purchaser, and I have no say when it comes to the artwork. When you're a porn star, you offer up your body for the viewing pleasure of so many, regardless of decorum or taste.

Exerting control in other areas of the industry has at times meant I've made choices that have ended up backfiring on me. My 'condom only' work, for instance, resulted in some good films with Wicked Pictures and VCA Pictures but caused too great a loss of income to support my working lifestyle. I eventually had to go back to doing condom-less shoots, and that backfired too, when I contracted chlamydia and gonorrhoea. There were only two occasions each when that happened, though – amazing given my output of more than 400 films over eight-plus years.

Around this time in my career, I was working on some great stuff, some really big-budget porn. (In porn, US$250,000 is big-budget.) For *Dark Angels 2: Bloodline*, shot in May 2005 for New Sensations, I sat with Nic Andrews, the director, and discussed vampires and fight scenes with him before he started production. I have always loved vampires and action scenes, so he thought I would be perfect for the role of Petra, the undead leading lady. I spent hours on my fight scene with a real Hollywood stunt coordinator, and my staged death was also pretty amazing, aided by computerised special effects. I think I should have won an award for acting and fucking in this movie, because the sex scene is unbelievable too (with Evan Stone, both of us as vampires performing wild, aggressive sex in the dark basement of an old downtown LA building). All of my friends who have watched my scenes in this movie are absolutely blown away. But hey, it's often about politics when it comes to winning awards.

A small role in *Sacred Sin* (Ninn Worx/Red Light District) came my way after that, which was still great because Michael Ninn is one of my favourite directors – he's so strangely creative and artistic. The film's music was scored by Eddie Van Halen, who was also its executive producer, and it went on to win Best Music, Best Art Direction and Best Videography at the 2007 AVN Awards. This was another US$250,000 big-budget production, and it was shot at Eddie's house. The first time I saw him, he was asleep on his couch with his guitar still in his hands. It was so cute. These stupid girls were being disrespectful and taking photos of him, but that image will always be in my head. Eddie's a freakin' legend, and an idol to most guitarists.

My sex scene itself was so crazy – me and Scott Nails on a pile of rocks, out in the freezing cold, with TV monitors all around us showing me enticing him to come and fuck me along with some other crazy images from the movie. Now, given that I was balancing on a pile of rocks, giving Scott a blow job and then having sex with him, I think I should also have been nominated for the AVN Best Sex Scene award. But meeting Eddie

Van Halen did mean I got to star in the music video for his song 'Rise'.

Professionally, 2005 was a very big year for me. That was the year that *Skin* was produced, and that is something I'm very proud of, for several reasons. Firstly, it was the movie for which I finally received my first nomination for an AVN award, for Best Solo Scene – for a scene where I'm masturbating in the shower. The film has no director's credit and it just says 'produced by Storm Productions' on the box-cover, but it was actually partly produced and directed by me and my friend Darren Kaye, who shoots mainly independent films. We distributed this movie through Skye Blue's then-company Platinum Blue (now defunct, as of November 2007); hence she is credited as executive producer. The film came out in 2006 but it was actually shot over a three-year period – 2003 to 2005 – which is why you'll see several scenes featuring me with my hair blonde and without tattoos and then others with my red hair and new tattoos. A number of things had kept getting in the way of its production – like finding an investor, and me being on the road so much that I didn't have time to do anything else.

Because I owned part of the movie, I decided it was the right place to perform my one-and-only anal scene, with my best friend Dez and his girlfriend, Alaura Eden. The three of us were all a bit drunk at the time and he challenged me to do it – 'C'mon, you tough Aussie!'

he kept taunting me – so I took him up on it. I can never resist a challenge. Several years later, when he was interviewed about doing my sole anal-sex scene with me, Dez said I did really well and it didn't even seem like that was my first-ever on-camera experience. 'She was great. She took it like a champ!' he said.

In the final cut of the movie, that whole three-way scene – me and Dez and Alaura making whoopee – is ridiculously long. It runs for 37 minutes in total, of which a whole nine minutes is yours truly getting frigged anally, my bare butt open wide for all to see. It was my idea to have completed footage from the actual movie play in the background – from my projector onto the wall behind us – while we were having sex, and I think it looks really great.

Dez, Alaura and I have had such good times together off-camera. There were many evenings where we'd meet at Taylor Rain's house – yes, we porn stars have our own house parties! – and our big thing was to play the computer simulation game *Rock Band* together. I got to play drums and break drumsticks, and it was always fun. I still relive those good memories in my mind and I know I'll always cherish them after I go home to Australia some day.

Another of my favourite movies that I shot around the same time as *Skin* was *Return to the Edge*, made for Adam & Eve in 2003. I was the lead in this fetish movie directed by Nick Orleans, set in a house with different fetish-themed rooms, in a swingers' party type of scenario. It remains memorable for a great glory-hole scene that I did with five guys. Their erections were the only things visible through open holes in the wall, and I took them each in my mouth, one at a time.

Steven St Croix was the male lead in that movie, and we used to shoot a lot together so I guess we had good on-set chemistry. But when he started seeing this new girl (whose name I won't mention), she got very jealous and ended up hating me. I finally confronted her about it at a party, and now we're friends. Anyway, a lot of acting was involved in this movie, which I always love, and the costumes were great. We got to wear some items from the film *Moulin Rouge*, so we had to be careful not to leave cum stains on the clothes!

In late 2005, I had an experience that changed my life. One evening, Dez called me up last minute to go with him to the Playboy Mansion. My friend Sky and I quickly got dressed and Dez picked us up in a limo. When we got there, a very well-known band was playing. Suddenly, Sky ripped off my dress and I was naked with all the other girls! That was not my intention, I'm not one of those girls who does that kind of thing, but I went with it. The lead guitarist came up to Sky and me after the show and said that his drummer was a big fan of Sky's, so we met up later that night and hung out in the grotto.

The next night, Sky went to the Teen Choice Awards with the drummer and while she was with him called me up to say that the guitarist wanted to see me. I couldn't remember what he looked like, as I had been pretty drunk at the Mansion. She reminded me he was cute, so I went to a bar, Dragonfly, in Hollywood to meet up with them. There was an instant connection – we were drawn to each other – and that never happens to me. We were dancing and making out when some fans of mine came up to me, some girls from Australia. I invited them back to his hotel room to party for a while, and they were calling up their boyfriends in Australia so I could say hi. It was hilarious. The guitarist was quite astonished and said to me, 'I can't believe I'm the rock star and *you* have the groupies!'

Eventually, I asked them to leave 'cause I wanted to be alone with this guy. After having deep conversations all night, we finally hooked up. I stayed all night and was kind of sad to see him go the next day.

When I look back over my journals from that time, I notice there are a lot of entries that are missing. I'm surprised, because my encounters with this guy over the last few years have been so dramatic, and I thought I would have recorded them. We fell in love and it was intense. It was like nothing I've ever experienced before. But circumstances and problems always kept us apart. It was never going to work. Long-distance relationships are tough, and we were on and off so many times. I even wrote a song about him called 'Never Again', which I think is one of the most beautiful songs I've ever written, although it makes me sad every time I hear it. I gave myself fully to this guy, but he just never believed I was for real.

And it seems now that I just can't fall for anyone else. I can't seem to let myself get attached to anyone. I really have major trust and abandonment issues. And guys have a really hard time trusting me too, because of what I do for a living.

It wasn't long after I fell for the rock star that I learned my mother had died. She had succumbed to cirrhosis of the liver – a common fate of dedicated drinkers – in November 2005. A few days beforehand, my aunt in England had emailed me to say my mother had lapsed into a coma. The morning I got the email saying she had finally died, I was supposed to go on a shoot. My initial reaction was, 'Wow, it's finally happened.'

I went to shoot a girl-on-girl scene like nothing had happened. My best friends Sky and Lisa came with me for moral support, in case I broke down or something, but I didn't. It was like a relief, actually. I didn't even cry. I knew this day would come, and I was already at peace with the fact that she would die soon, so I wasn't going to put my life on hold just to sit around and think about it all day. All my life, I'd been kept repressed and restricted by her, so now that she was well and truly gone I was going to do what I wanted to do, all the way. So what if I was shooting porn? She had indirectly put me there.

My brother, on the other hand, had a very different situation to deal with. When my mother died, she didn't have a funeral and had already requested that she should be cremated and her ashes sent to Wales, to be sprinkled over her beloved homeland. My poor brother, being the eldest sibling, had to take care of it and it was extraordinarily difficult for him, since he despised her. I used to hear her beating him in the hallway at night when I was younger, and I remember how I would push my bed up against the door so she couldn't come into my room to do the same for me. I literally would be shaking and crying in my room, afraid to go to sleep, thinking she was possessed by some demon.

I don't think my brother ever got over what she did to us, yet he had to spend a lot of his own money sorting out her stuff and arranging for the cremation. The irony was that she had inherited a lot of money after her own mother had died, but as usual she'd spent it on her own good self – on expensive vacations she paid for but never took, and on cruises she did take but didn't complete because they booted her off the ships for drunken behaviour.

She had also donated AU$50,000 to the Red Cross and to the Hurricane Katrina rescue fund just a couple of months before she died. Her acts of whimsical philanthropy were gleefully offset by her warning to us that she would cut us out of her will if we didn't call her on command or do whatever she said. That was her in a nutshell – bitter to the end. I still like to think that the money went to a good cause, since it sure didn't go to us.

With my mother's death, I felt as though a huge weight had been lifted off my shoulders. She was a hard, miserable woman who hated herself and hated life, and now she was finally at peace. I always felt sorry for her, even when we were fighting. I knew deep down that she was being difficult because she could never be happy. She tried to kill herself six times, after all.

To this day, I'm still somewhat resentful of the fact that my mum never encouraged me to do the things I wanted to do. She turned down every opportunity that came my way whenever people wanted me to sing or act, and I think that she was jealous of me because she wanted so badly to be in the spotlight herself. Whenever I told her I wanted to pursue a career in music, she would say, 'Yeah, right.' She constantly put me down and laughed at me, even in her later years.

The last time I saw her was when I tried to make amends by visiting her where she was living in Tasmania, a couple of years before she died. I'd told her about my career by this time, but I think it had gone in one ear and out the other. She didn't even care what I was doing, and I don't think she ever comprehended that I was a porn star. On this last occasion, she actually had the gall to say to me, 'It hasn't been a very good life for you, has it?' Now, how's that for twisting the knife? She was the one who had basically ensured that my life hadn't been a bed of roses and now she was rubbing it in my face!

So, that's how it ended for my mum and me, in Tasmania. I cried and told her, 'You know what? I now realise that nothing ever changes, and so I just came here to say goodbye.'

However, on looking back, I realise I do have something to thank her for: getting me out of Kenmore. Had I not fought her torrent of abuse, I might never have left and my life to date might never have happened.

Chapter Seven

COMPILATIONS AND VIOLATIONS

One of the many strange things about porn is that once you're done filming, you have no way to know how your work will be packaged, marketed or received. While it is good to know that what you've done has brought pleasure to people, even if they're expressing their appreciation by masturbating furiously to your image, they don't have a clue at all about who you really are or what you're like as a person, because they're fixating on you as a sex symbol. Which is all well and good, since that's the job I'm supposed to do, the function I'm paid to fulfil. But it is difficult to accept that, most of the time, scenes I shoot could end up anywhere – on the internet or on a compilation – and I won't get any more money for that.

Compilations are a thorny issue to us girls because we know that the companies have the right to re-use scenes shot for certain movies and slap them into 'new' movies – akin to how record companies release 'greatest hits' compilations for their recording artists (especially when their contracts expire, so that the company can make more money out of existing material). Unlike recording artists, though, we don't get paid residuals or anything extra for these additional 'movies' and there's just nothing we can do about it, because we don't have any kind of unionised collective bargaining in porn and nobody sticks up for our rights.

I once did a scene in a movie for my ex-husband, Craven, called *Bustin' Nuts on Sluts*, which had a really great box-cover, but I found out later that he used that *same* scene (and the cover *too*) for a 'new' movie called *Fuck Me Like the Whore That I Am*. (Yep, that's a typical Craven comment. That's really what he thought of me!) This kind of recycling happens all the time in porn. And nobody cares if you get called a whore, because it's supposed to be funny.

Anabolic Video did the same thing to porn star Sabrina Johnson, a really lovely English girl, back in 1999, when they strung together two hours of her scenes into a compilation called *A Cum Sucking Whore Named Sabrina*, along with this riveting piece of box-cover copy:

Anabolic brings you a collection of scenes of a Brit whose main source of food just may be the salty semen that shoots from the work that her pimp/husband finds her! We believe her primary source of income is to suck, fuck or do whatever else he might tell her to, to whomever he tells her to! Thus, *A Cum Sucking Whore Named Sabrina*! Enjoy!

Now, that might sound funny in a porn-friendly ironic way, but to those in the know, it had a weird subtext. Sabrina's real-life husband, Graham, had actually been busted and jailed for nine months for 'living off immoral earnings', so these guys at Anabolic were deliberately cashing in on the couple's notoriety. It's sometimes hard to say what's ethically or morally correct when it comes to an entire industry that deals in dubious interpretations and grey areas all the time. I know that if I was Sabrina, I doubt I would find that at all funny.

This kind of marketing feeds straight into the judgemental mindset of all those people who'll adopt the posture of moral rectitude and use it to condemn girls like Sabrina and myself. And I think that attitude sucks.

Just because we play sexually voracious women in our movies, does that automatically mean that we are equally accepting of what gets done to us by those who deem us lower than we deserve? In other words, do we deserve to be treated like whores just because we play those parts? And why should any woman be demeaned just because she is a whore, or because she stays close to her 'inner slut' (as progressive, pro-porn feminists have argued) and isn't ashamed of expressing herself with her body?

Which leads me to the second example, one that for me is much closer to the bone (pardon the innuendo). In October 2007, I learned that my one and only anal sex scene in the movie *Skin* had been used again, without my prior knowledge, in a compilation film about anal sex called *The Ass Hammer*. Both films were released by Platinum Blue, but *Skin* was funded by an investor, and part of the contract was that they would not use any of the footage in any other films. Yet here they were doing exactly that. They also used still photos from *Skin*, which is a breach of contract too.

Unfortunately for me, Platinum Blue went belly-up a month later, leaving my investor and me high and dry. Neither of us has been paid as much as a single cent for either of these films to this day, and we don't expect to recoup our losses any time soon, since there's nobody to collect from, given the financial insolvency of the distribution company. I was well and truly fucked, in the very real sense of that word, and I was well and truly pissed off.

I was initially so proud of *Skin*, but my enthusiasm soured after I found out how they'd used my anal sex scene in this way. It made me look bad to the buying public, because I now appeared to have not just one but two anal scenes out there, even though it was the very same scene. How was I supposed to correct this misperception in the marketplace? And how was I to appease some of my fans who might recognise the recycling of that scene and feel disappointed, because it now looked like I was out to make more money any way I could, even though this kind of avaricious behaviour was not my own doing at all?

I contacted one of the producers of *The Ass Hammer*, who I'd thought until then was a personal friend, and he said I should have known better and that they had every right to use anything they wanted for compilation movies, which was bullshit. 'Wow,' I thought, 'some kind of friend you are, mate!'

To this day, that whole debacle remains unresolved. A friend of a friend lost his life savings because of that whole mess. I felt bad for referring this guy to Platinum Blue, but I had no idea we were going to get ripped off. And, really, I didn't force him to take the offer – we could've shopped it around some more, but he too thought it was a great deal and decided to take a chance.

I learned a very valuable lesson from that whole sordid saga: just because you enjoy being sexually objectified, doesn't mean there aren't people out there who won't use that to their own advantage and for their own monetary gain, like putting your scenes in comps without your knowledge, much less your approval, or selling your images to websites or for phone sex ads.

Controlling your photographic image is just as difficult as controlling the use of your sex scenes. A free newspaper called the *LA Xpress* had me on their cover once, which I initially didn't mind because it was really an advertorial photo featuring the VCA logo (since I'd shot a bunch of movies for VCA, so I saw it as free publicity for me). I found out later that the *LA Xpress* was a paper advertising sexual services of all kinds, mostly for 'healing' and 'therapy' by hookers. The cover shot had the unfortunate side effect of generating interest in me of a totally unexpected and unwanted kind – my name and photo ended up being used on several escorting websites, none of which I have any actual association with, and I have no legal recourse to have these photos removed. There are just too many of them – one of the very real downsides of instant publishing via the internet!

Times have definitely changed in the adult-film industry since I began in 2001. I used to get so many more lead-actress roles – more so than any contract girl. I was getting so much great work to do, and so much money, that for a lot of my career I thought a contract wasn't necessary. Now I realise it would've helped me to have been under contract more, since people seem to care so much about the 'contract girl' label these days.

Just like in the old Hollywood studio system, the adult-film industry likes to sign up girls on contracts whereby they have exclusive rights to film them in a certain number of movies over a certain period of time – usually a year – turning them into stars along the way by giving them major publicity and exposure. Vivid Girls are a good example of this, as they seem to have a certain prestige.

Because I'm not a contract girl, it seems like I don't get as much respect as I used to, even though my name on a box-cover will sell a lot of movies. I found that out from Adam & Eve and VCA, two companies for whom I've shot a lot of lead roles. They both offered me contracts, but VCA's offer was very small, and I would have accepted the Adam & Eve contract except after they made the offer they changed management and withdrew it, despite saying they would be able to sell at least 5000 units of my movies right off the bat, which was huge.

These days, contract-girl status is something all porn stars are supposed to covet, and what the fans all believe to be the ultimate validation of our worth as porn stars. It sounds so glamorous and, in theory, it is. What girl wouldn't want that? The freedom to work on only a specified number of films each year for an agreed amount of money that is guaranteed income sounds pretty good, right?

The idea is sound on paper, provided you read your contract and sign off on what you believe to be a win–win situation. The downsides, though, can be that the company 'owns' you and tells you what you can and can't do, including not changing your hair, not getting tattoos, not doing any shoots or interviews or attending events that they don't approve of, and they can also own your website and your name, which they may not give back to you after the contract expires.

From the viewpoint of us performers, it might save us from the plight of the freelance girl who has to schlep from shoot to shoot, making her money where she can, but reality can also bite hard. There have been a lot of contract girls at every company who have left their contracts without renewing them or found themselves abandoned by those very companies that originally wanted them, for all kinds of reasons.

I've only ever signed one contract-girl agreement, and that was with Cherry Boxxx Pictures. The year was 2003, and I was optimistic because Cherry Boxxx were new at the time and I believed they were going to become a big-name company. I took a chance and came on board. The deal was sound when I accepted it, since it meant I was locked into a non-exclusive arrangement for six movies for a year.

The most notable (and, I believe, the best-selling) movie that emerged from this deal was *Monica's Sex Crimes*. Rick Davis, the director, knew I wanted creative input in every movie I did with them so he allowed me to pitch this idea: I'm a girlfriend of a mob boss who hands out rewards to his employees who have done a good job. I either hook them up with a hot chick or have sex with them myself as payment for their good work. I did three hot scenes: one with Cheyne Collins, one with a sexy Latino named Sergio and one with a sexy brunette from Scarborough, New York, named Venus. (She was my own reward for doing such a good job for the boss's hitmen!) We shot for 12 hours and I was doing dialogue in every scene, plus doing my own hair and make-up. I even posed for the box-cover that day. I was seriously ill with the worst cold ever on the day of the shoot but I still showed up to work because I didn't want to cost them money by cancelling. The funny thing is that when I watched the movie, I didn't even look sick. It was one of Cherry Boxxx's biggest sellers, and I was *almost* nominated for an AVN award – I got a pre-nomination for Best Sex Scene.

However, there were a couple of hitches in my time as a contract girl. One of them had nothing to do with the shoots, and it was really a fucked-up situation. While I was at the AVN convention, signing autographs for Cherry Boxxx, the company publicist kept pulling me aside to do interviews to promote the company, so half my days were spent signing autographs for my fans and the other half were spent doing these interviews. Fine, I thought, I can juggle my schedule to accommodate this schizoid plan, so I agreed to it.

But a sales lady who worked there, who just hated me, told the boss that I was hardly ever at the signing booth. When I got back to LA and was paid, I discovered that they'd docked US$500 from my cheque – because, they told me, I 'wasn't there the whole time'. I explained I was doing interviews for their company, but apparently that didn't count for anything.

I was left to conclude that being devoted to a company, helping them to make money, was *not* a good way to do business. At the time, I was thinking I could do with some extra publicity, but what good is publicity when you're not benefiting financially from it? (A lesson learned, and a warning to all you new girls!)

It's no coincidence, by the way, that in this business many girls get their contracts while dating certain directors or owners of companies. I put my hand up to dating the owner of Cherry Boxxx, but only *after* I had obtained my contract and had already shot two films. When people ask me what the heck happened with my Cherry Boxxx contract, I tell them, 'My contract was up, and I moved on.'

I could be bitter about all this now, but I really have no animosity to either Cherry Boxxx or to the boss. The years have passed and I've got on with my career. I have worked for Rick Davis again a couple of times since I left my Cherry Boxxx contract, and in 2008 I shot my movie *Rockstar Pornstar* for the Cherry Boxxx owner's new company, Sex Line Sinema. It's all part of being professional about it, and I try not to bear grudges – especially if they impede my mission to get more work!

Was it a bad idea to date the owner of the company I was signed to? Well, at least one good thing came from it, and that was while I was with him he made sure

I did only girl–girl scenes. (Hmm, why are guys who date porn stars always so jealous that they want us to work only with girls and not other men? Having sex with another guy for work is just too real for them, I guess.) This had a fortunate unforeseen consequence – when the HIV scare of 2004 broke and several girls were infected, I was spared, since I hadn't had sex with men for work. Boy, was I lucky!

Not everybody likes to admit it, but the porn industry is about taking the money and running these days, for all involved. The fun has gone and the work itself is like clockwork now. There's definitely a mechanical aspect to it: like doing any job, you have a routine and a method. Once you're on a roll, once you know you're good and it's working, you just go in and do the same thing each time. When you've done it that many times, you just want to be professional, get it done and get through the shoot as quickly as possible. Why waste time waiting for the photographer to tell you what to do when you already know?

I think I have definitely learned all I needed to learn out of porn. I've seen everything and I've done everything that I've wanted to do. I don't need to do anything more. I think the industry has helped me, too, because I didn't have much self-esteem going into it and now I do feel more confident about a lot of things. I am still not a hundred per cent secure in myself, but I am a lot better than I used to be.

I was so innocent when I started out, but once you've done it a lot it becomes part of your everyday life, so it's nothing to me now and I don't think twice about shooting a scene. That's what people mean when they tell me 'You're a legend', even though I never came into this industry wanting to be a legend. I just came here thinking I was going to make some money and leave. Next thing you know, it's really hard to quit.

As I've said, I didn't really know anything about porn before entering the business, so I didn't realise I was entering the industry at the end of an era, when the gonzo craze was about to hit. I think I only noticed this when the work for features slowed down and many directors started telling me they thought I was 'too good for gonzo'. They were reluctant to hire me or even *ask* me if I wanted to shoot, because they thought my rates were sky-high or that I would turn them down. (I mean, is it my fault that I can actually do dialogue?)

All I had really done was feature films, and I thought maybe gonzo was just really nasty stuff so I didn't need it anyway, when it turns out that it's more just constant hardcore action (with no softcore for the TV market), no, or next to no, storyline and, of course, no script.

Perhaps as a consequence, and also because it's cheaper, the directors in porn these days are seldom interested in your acting skills – a couple of takes is usually good enough, and you're not really given enough time to get into character properly, especially with no real rehearsals and often no real direction. I really miss the days when I had to learn my script and shoot dialogue scenes or action/stunt scenes. I didn't care how many 14-hour days it took. I was so happy just to be *acting* in any way, shape or form, because that's what I really love to do. It kills me to not be doing that as much now, with the industry going through its severe downturn.

Another thing I have had to learn to accept as a porn star is the sheer inevitable time-crunch of my publicity obligations. Sometimes, I don't really want to spend my whole day doing something that's purely a promotional exercise but I know that in the long run it will be good for me. Getting my name out there is what the game is about, if you want to be a professional.

Not everyone in the industry behaves as professionally as I do, though. I've shot with many photographers who didn't pay much and weren't the easiest guys to get along with. It's very frustrating when they're yelling at you to do something that is physically impossible, or when the person paying for the shoot wants to control everything. For example, I was shooting a billboard for a strip club in LA, and not only was the guy so cheap that he hired a food photographer – to shoot for free – but he also wanted creative control of everything, including me!

I can't stand it when people at these shoots are too hands-on, trying to move me into position rather than

Absolute Mayhem

just telling me what they want. But this club owner thought he could just fling me around, pulling my arms in different directions, all the while having no clue what he was doing. I was not impressed at all.

Another, much more famous, photographer I have worked with thinks he's the shit, like he's the best photographer in the world. He'll even tell you that to your face, if you can believe such arrogance. This guy didn't even shoot me but had his assistant do it while he was doing something else in the other room. He'll pay each girl US$400 or US$500 and they have to put up with his crap. I heard from one girl that he got her to hold a pose and while she was doing it, not moving a muscle, he just left the room and went out to lunch and didn't come back. What an asshole!

And it's not just the photographers who can be temperamental. Sometimes, your fellow porn stars can be just as bad. A well-known male porn star and I used to work together frequently because we had great on-screen chemistry. We had shot a lot of scenes and he was always on my top-five list, until one day he totally screwed me over.

After shooting with me the night before, he ran into me at the doctor's office, where either he or his girlfriend were being treated for gonorrhoea. I had never had the disease at that stage, but nevertheless he called the director and told him that I had given it to him. He said that I knew I had it and was going to work anyway. I was at the doctor's for something totally unrelated to that, but he just assumed I was there to get tested or treated for gonorrhoea, and he made me look like a scumbag.

So the director cancelled my scene for the next day and said I should get tested – which I did, and I was clean. I sorted things out with the director and eventually finished the movie, but I will never forgive this guy for doing that. He also told that story to many people, when it was just not true.

That's just a reality check for some girls who think this is all about glitz and glamour. And here's another: leaning back against a couch and keeping still while you're holding your vagina wide open for a still camera, waiting for the close-up to happen and praying your last shave will look good – that's not a regular day at the office for most girls, but it sure is to me.

You do have to be mindful of the mind-fuck, so to speak, when you get to my level. For instance, when I do live chats on the IM Live site (www.imlive.com), I get my share of strange requests from the fans. There's the usual boob-licking, pussy-squirting and foot-fetish stuff, but I also get asked to consider doing pissing and scatting – guys wanting me to say 'I want you to eat my shit' and one guy who said he likes shit on his belly and balls so he can fuck it back into the girl.

I also get asked about using my panties. One guy said he only wanted to buy them if I stuffed them inside my pussy first! (I mean, how the hell do you stuff your own panties inside you? How painful is that?) I also get asked to simulate cum in my mouth – these guys like me to put my mouth to the webcam and use my spit to pretend it's their cum. Oh boy.

But, of course, I can't or won't always cater to what everyone wants, especially the rude fucks who are just plain demanding. Instead of asking me to do something, they seem to think they can tell me what to do, like I am some stupid whore stuck in a cage or something. If I'm not comfortable doing something, I simply won't do it. That's just how I work, even though some people don't seem to understand that.

The crazy sex is definitely not confined to the internet. In August 2008, I shot one of my strangest scenes when Jim Powers directed me in *The Violation of Harmony*, for JM Productions. Basically, the plot was like *America's Next Top Model*. We were the contestants, and the porn star Harmony was the Tyra Banks character, only white. She was a total bitch to all of us and had pushed us too far, so we turned on her and raped her. It took all day to shoot and I was really exhausted in the end. Being mean really takes a lot out of you! The girls were Audrey Hollander, Summer Bailey, Holly Wellin, Jennifer Dark and me. It was a really wild shoot because Harmony was a chick who could take anything! She was very loose (if I can use that adjective as a compliment), because we were sticking huge toys in her, double-penetrating her and sometimes sticking two sex toys in her pussy and one in her ass simultaneously. We were holding her down, smacking her face and even sticking our dirty feet in her mouth and making her lick them. We were calling her names and telling her what a fat whore she was. It was brutal.

Jim Powers was good to work with as a director. He's very cool and a bit of a smartass, and somewhat perverted. At one point, he had me stick my foot inside Harmony's vagina. I mean, I actually had my *whole* foot in this chick, up to my ankle. It felt pretty disgusting and gross, to be honest, because it's just not normal to have your foot in such a place. And I'd always thought of myself as a girl who didn't pussyfoot around!

I can take perversions, believe me, but we all have our limits. Jim Powers was Walt Disney compared to some other directors I've worked for, like Martin Del Toro, who really loves shooting rough sex with women.

I did a blow-bang scene for him once in which I sucked off five guys. Quite appropriately, the movie was entitled *Cum Greed*, and it was released in 2005 by VCA. They were all really rough with me, grabbing my head and pulling my hair and ramming their cocks down my throat, because that's what Martin, as the director calling the shots, wanted. Most of the guys felt bad, I could tell, but one of them loved doing it, from the way he grabbed and manhandled me.

Sure, I can do this stuff, and I'm game for extreme sex, but it was a really rough scene and in the end I felt so degraded. I had make-up running all down my face, and the scene had climaxed with all of them ejaculating on me. Not all over my face or my breasts, bukkake-style, but rather each one of them took turns to shoot his sperm right into my mouth. Then I had to spit it out onto the camera lens and slurp it all back up, before spitting it out again. It was seriously nasty work.

On another occasion, I also had to pee into a guy's mouth. The actor was Alec Metro and I stood over him for ten minutes before I could expel any urine. I eventually peed right into Alec's mouth and he actually gargled it before swallowing. I was grossed out. I mean, this was *before* our sex scene, so I was doing this glorious act of urophilia to a man I then had to have sex with. I have no idea why anyone would even want to see such a thing.

So, I'll challenge anyone to tell me if they've encountered weirder ways of making money. What we girls get paid is often not at all commensurate with the head-trip we have to endure to play those parts. It's amazing to me when all these teenage girls come up to me and say they want to become porn stars because they are nymphomaniacs and think it is just so glamorous. Little do they know, especially about the fine line between exhibitionism and exploitation. I do understand how some guys enjoy looking at girls who behave like total sluts, but it can sometimes get downright tasteless.

There are times when even I am stunned by how absurd this profession is. It's literally a dirty job, and someone has got to do it. I've had to shoot scenes with guys I used to date. Imagine having to fuck someone you broke up with, because you're getting paid to do it! In one case, a porn-star ex-boyfriend of mine called Barrett Blade hadn't worked with me for at least four years. It was great in the end, but I'm sure we were both thinking the same thing while the cameras were rolling. It was actually kind of a turn-on for both of us, as it turned out. You could ration-alise it and remind yourself that, well, at least you already *know* the guy, when in fact, really, it's just too surreal.

I've also had to do scenes with guys and girls whom I didn't particularly like as people, as well as those with whom I had great sex but who stabbed me in the back afterwards. For the legion of nymphettes scouring the San Fernando Valley for work every week, these kinds of scenarios will become part of their bread-and-butter month after month, year after year.

There's a lot more to this job than its just being well-paid work for any exhibitionist who loves sex. It has always been my own personal belief that you have to be truly, uniquely courageous to stay the course. You become a commodity, something to be bought and sold like a box of cereal on a shelf. There are people within the industry who will keep treating you like this. And sexual harassment on the job does happen, however ironic that must sound.

I can honestly say I have never gone so far as to do anything for anyone just to get a role. I do remember one incident, though, back when I was very new to the industry. A very well-known director asked me if I wanted to go to an audition at his house at around 9 pm. I mean, come on. Who holds auditions at their house at night? The studio he was directing movies for already held huge castings all the time at their offices during the day. I wasn't that naive. So, of course, I said no. And the result? He never once put me in any of his movies, not even to this very day.

Chapter Eight

HEALTH BEFORE WEALTH

The first time you see me in the 'Behind the Scenes' section of *Dark Angels 2: Bloodline*, my personal favourite of all my films, it isn't the part where I'm flexing my legs and practising my kick-boxing stunts. Neither is it my rehearsals of the fight scene with Dillon Day where he's on the ground and I attack him from above, which we went over again and again while trying not to laugh. It is the part where I'm bending over, trying to do some warm-up callisthenics and yoga stretching exercises. Why? Because they could point the camera straight at my ass and shoot me from behind. But, in all seriousness, warming up and stretching are very important parts of my job.

To survive this business, you have to take care of your well-being. I am quite a believer in the holistic mind–body relationship, and I do think that a sound mind needs to go with a sound body. This industry constantly poses challenges to that equation. I can barely count the weird things I have had to deal with now, because there have been way too many to recall, but let me cite a few.

Back when I started out, when Roy Garcia was my agent, I did a shoot for a Japanese company. I was brand new and willing to try pretty much anything. A Japanese company came into town with some famous Japanese male porn star (and a translator, because none of them spoke English). We started the scene off like a typical gonzo shoot – no plot, no script – and then suddenly they're yelling at me to scream louder.

So I thought, 'Okay, they want me to highly exagger-ate it.'

I did the loud moans and groans, and then they were like, 'No, louder!' So I did it louder. And again, 'Louder!'

At that point, I stopped and said, 'Look, are you fucking serious? I'm moaning as loud as I can!'

The translator pulled me aside and told me that the Japanese get off on the appearance of a girl getting raped. So they actually wanted me to scream like I was terrified, like I was being raped. And he wasn't kidding. That's what they wanted. I was not comfortable with this at all. I didn't sign up to be 'raped', nor did I want to act like I was, and I thought the whole thing was really twisted. So I did the best I could do. I realise I could have just acted and screamed like crazy, but it just didn't seem right to me. Apparently, they were not happy with my performance at all. But who cares? I wasn't happy with the way I was treated. How was I supposed to fake being raped like I was enjoying it?

I know this is a very real phenomenon in Japanese porn – the prevailing theory is that Japanese men are brought up by very strict mothers and use porn to channel their resentment of women – so we had a real culture clash there.

On another occasion, I found myself sought after for yet another Japanese scenario. This shoot would entail me spending an hour kicking a guy in the nuts really hard and then jerking him off to pop – a quickie scene for US$500. When it was offered to me, I thought, 'Hmm, wouldn't that be hilarious, to kick a guy in the nuts?'

Later, I learned that the Japanese have a whole sub-genre of porn dedicated to this, which even has a name – *tamakeri* (which, loosely translated, means 'ball-kicking'). There are female porn stars in Japan, like Erika Nagai, who specialise in it, and there are even ground rules to be observed (yes, *tamakeri* etiquette). The male actor has to maintain his erection during and after he is being kicked, and the girl is supposed to kick him as hard as possible so that a loud, slapping sound can be heard. Japanese social scientists have studied *tamakeri,* and one of them, Nobuhiro Hashimoto, believes it's due to the 'latent masochism' in Japanese male culture – the kind of thing that's also exemplified by other kinds of Japanese porn, like scenes featuring the opposite of a gang-bang, where a bunch of hot Japanese babes take turns urinating on a helpless guy, and those where the girls, after pissing, take turns excreting on the guy! Japanese guys really get off on this kind of shit? I'm not sure I'd venture any further than *tamakeri,* thank you.

I did once work on an anime porn project, using my voice for the English version of the soundtrack. The film was called *Kokudu-oh* and it was a lot of fun to record. I love doing voice-over work and would like to do more of it. In this particular anime (or, more precisely, *hentai,* as animated porn is called in Japan), I voiced Princess Bellecher, a very sexy blonde virgin princess, with (of course) huge boobs. There was a prince and another girl (voiced by Aria Giovanni) and the whole thing consisted of four episodes.

The storyline has the prince looking for a wife to become the queen of the kingdom. In one scene, he rapes Princess Bellecher in a jacuzzi and the tub fills up with blood, and I had to make the funniest noises to kind of make it sound like the Japanese version. Another scene had him locking Princess Bellecher up in a room before tying her nipples to the floor so that every time she tried to move, she would be in great pain. And he also gives her an enema at one point. There was a lot of raping and sexual abuse going on in that movie – just the way they like it in Japan.

We were recording my voice to sell the film to an American fan base, but I don't think it did very well over here, because the company went broke. When I had to sign autographs for it at a comic convention in Long Beach, though, the comic fans went absolutely nuts. They love these *hentai* movies – and the queues were even longer than the ones I've dealt with signing for real porn fans at the AVN Expo!

How do I do this kind of work at all, you might well ask, and what does it do to my head? On the simplest level, all porn stars know that we have to perform blow jobs while we're being filmed, and that alone is a mental Zen exercise. There's a lot of gobbling in porn, so if you don't like taking a penis in your mouth you can't be a porn star – there's no two ways around that. But there are a lot of issues you have to be mentally prepared for.

For starters, you have to find different ways to pleasure a guy orally, and the girls who are good at it know all the tricks – using saliva, sucking his balls and then his shaft and going back and forth on that, using one hand to stroke and sometimes both hands to rotate the area around the shaft – but there are times when you've got to work five times as hard for the same result.

And then there is the whole issue with swallowing sperm. Some girls really get neurotic about this but

I don't have a problem with it at all. In real life, I like swallowing if I like the guy I'm with. For a movie, I'll swallow if I'm directed to do so. It doesn't matter who the guy is, really.

What I don't like is getting cum in my eyes. I remember one shoot where I was told I was going to be doing a threesome. I wasn't told the names of the girl and the guy or anything before I arrived and actually met them, and when I did they were strangers to me. (Isn't that amazing? Going to work, not knowing whom you're going to be fucking, only that you will be?) Anyway, the truth is I like doing threesomes. I don't mean necessarily in real life, but when it's for a movie. The reason is clear after you've worked like I have for a while. Because you're doing two positions each – two on the girl and two on the guy, instead of four positions on just one guy – it's so much easier on your body.

The shoot turned out to be quite long, but it was pretty good. The girl had big titties, which I love. The guy who was scheduled for our scene bailed out because he had girlfriend drama (how lame!) so we got a production assistant from the crew to do it. Lucky guy, huh? He was awesome and had a nice cock. It was his second scene ever, and he came all over our faces when it was supposed to be only from the chin down. He just couldn't control it. It was a real 'Peter North' pop shot, as we call it (named after the male porn stud famous for his 'beer can' ejaculations). But I was not happy about getting cum in my eye. It was still throbbing after the shoot and I had to cancel a live chat session for my website that night. Damn it! Did anyone ever warn me about the occupational hazard of getting cum in my eye? Of course not.

There have been times when I've felt like the guy had too much control over me when I was sucking him, and that I was giving away too much of myself. Lots of guys just want you to suck it because it's an ego trip for them. In my personal life, if I sense that they're just being a selfish prick, I won't always give them the satisfaction (simply because I know I do it pretty well, and they need to earn that privilege from me).

When all you have to do is a blow-job scene and you don't have to have penetrative sex with the guy, giving good head is an excellent way of performing to get quick cash. This is truly a win–win situation if the guy I have to be with happens to have a very large cock.

For any girl, huge cocks can really be a source of pain. Quite a few guys in the industry are hung like horses and some girls seem to love this – usually because they are loose enough to take it – but not me, since I'm very small down there. When I've done a scene that has been particularly painful, I like to use an ice pack between my legs and try not to have sex or touch that area until the next time I have to work or until it stops hurting, whichever comes first.

Anal sex is a different matter. As you know, I've only ever done one anal scene on-camera. I could have made US$5000 for other anal sex scenes, which was what a lot of directors were offering me, but I thought I was being smart owning my own anal scene. Oh well. The main thing about preparing for anal sex is adjusting your headspace. It helps if you've done it in real life, so that you've tried it before doing it in front of a camera. And you *must* like it a little bit. Some girls love it (or say they love it) but I'm honest enough to admit that it was really uncomfortable for me.

Before shooting an anal-sex scene, you need to do an enema beforehand to clean yourself out. Don't eat and definitely drink no coffee and use no laxatives before the shoot – you don't want any messy accidents! And just relax. (Ah, isn't that the hard part?) If the guy doesn't know how to do anal, you're in trouble. They need to ease it in, because there are three layers to penetrate, and once you get past that third layer, it's not so bad. For myself, however, I'd say give me plain and simple vaginal intercourse any time (although there *have* been a few occasions in my private life, I admit, where I'll have a mood swing while having sex and yell out, 'Put it in my ass!').

So, while we're still in that area, let me share something with you that you might be wondering about: how do porn stars get their assholes so clean shaven and good looking? The comedian Sarah Silverman wrote an

138

article for the December 1999 issue of *Penthouse* called 'Thank Heaven for Penthouse Pets' in which she said that the first and foremost reason why she admires them is because 'Penthouse Pets wax their assholes. Right there, you gotta respect that. For that, they deserve the Purple Heart. I don't have the guts to wax my asshole, and neither do you.'

That's pretty funny, but I'll tell you for the record that I've never waxed my asshole. But I do have my own foolproof method. I do it only when I have to shoot, and it's the most pain-in-the-ass fucking procedure. First of all, you can do it in your bathtub or in the shower, but you must not have the water running on you. You have to squat down and get there from underneath – I'll put one leg up, spread a cheek, bend over and shave, and then do the other side, put the other leg up, bend over and shave. It's really, really difficult and you have to be a contortionist. I'm not into waxing – it's not a good idea to get that area waxed because you might tear something – and I don't know any other way. I think some girls do wax and some girls just don't get hair growing there, so they're just lucky. It's really, really irritating, trying to shave your own asshole – now there's another occupational hazard! It is very easy to nick yourself. That's happened to me, though nothing bad, and it occurred when I was rushing it.

As for my vagina, I don't like being fully shaved. I like leaving a tiny strip of hair – which we call the 'landing strip'. (When I'm fully shaved, like I have to be on some shoots, I feel like I'm a baby or a 12-year-old.) As I've already confessed, when I first started I didn't really know what I needed to do. I didn't even know that you had to shave around your vaginal lips and everything. But I learned pretty fast that girls don't like it much when they have to work with other girls who are really bushy down there, because of getting all that hair in their mouths. It's unhygienic and doesn't do anything for anyone.

I shave my vagina every day when I'm shooting, or as often as necessary when I'm not. Sometimes, you'll get an uncomfortable rash if you don't shave for a few days. I use a vibrating Gillette Venus. I never cut myself there, and when I shave in the shower it can be quite fun.

In my line of work, whether you perform anal or not, there's the constant exposure to STDs. I get myself tested every 28 days, and I've always gone through Adult Industry Medical (AIM) Healthcare in Sherman Oaks, the excellent facility started by former porn star Sharon Mitchell and her friend Dr Stephen York. It was founded in 1998 to help sex workers get themselves tested regularly and has two locations in Southern California (in Sherman Oaks and Granada Hills). Sharon herself has a PhD in human sexuality and is very active, both in the medical community and as the industry's de facto spokesperson to the press whenever an AIDS or HIV scare occurs. I've asked my doctor how much it would cost to get my tests done through their clinic every month, and it would be US$350, as opposed to AIM, which charges US$120 per month.

I readily give praise to AIM for how they handled things with the last big HIV scare, back in April 2004. They put up degrees-of-separation charts, listing the people who directly came into contact with the HIV source, then the people who were at one remove from it, two removes from it, etc., etc. This was the time when the owner of Cherry Boxxx Pictures had me doing only girl–girl scenes, of course, so my risks of getting it were greatly reduced. It was such a scary period, nevertheless. It was due to a guy named Darren James, then a performer for seven years, who had gone to Brazil to shoot and came back infected with the HIV virus. I remember that when I was married to Craven and he once told me he was going to Brazil to shoot, I begged him to use condoms. 'Whatever you do, whoever you fuck, *please* wear a condom,' I told him, and he just laughed at me. I'd heard that the porn stars over there could get a fake clean test for just US$10.

Anyway, as the story goes, Darren James shot a bunch of scenes down there for two weeks and came back to LA with his test still current. He then shot a bunch of scenes without getting re-tested – after shooting in a foreign country, which is a big no-no. His test was still only two weeks old, not 28 days yet, and he went ahead and did a gang-bang and a bunch of anal-cream-pie scenes (when the guy ejaculates inside the girl's ass

and the camera captures his sperm oozing out of her) –
not knowing that he had already contracted HIV from
some Brazilian porn chick.

Twelve girls were involved with Darren and his circle,
and that's how the virus began to spread. Jessica Dee and
Lara Roxx were the first to be named among the infected.
Jessica, from the Czech Republic, was then 25 years old
and, luckily for her, Platinum X co-owner Jewel De'Nyle
then hired her as a director so she could work behind the
camera instead. Lara, from Montreal, Canada, was only
21 years old at the time and had been working in porn for
just three months. She moved back to Montreal shortly
after the outbreak and said in an interview on *Entertainment Tonight* that she had regrets about her short stay
in porn. 'I was just pretending to be happy about it,' she
reflected. 'I thought US$2000 a day sounded attractive.
I expected that I could go sleep with whoever I wanted
and I thought that the actresses ruled.' Now, she was
afraid of 'dying too early, too soon, too young'.

I remember feeling terrified – because a lot of my
friends and some guys that I had always preferred to
work with were on those long HIV-generation lists,
which went on and on and made everyone paranoid. It
felt so surreal, like the end of the world. There were so
many obvious questions being asked, like 'How could
this have happened?' and 'How can we prevent this from
happening in the future?', and I really felt like quitting
the business at that point.

The mainstream press, of course, got great mileage out of it. *The New York Times* ran a piece on 17 April 2004 with the headline 'HIV Case Shuts Down Pornographic Film Industry', documenting how an entire industry that churned out 4000 films a year had to stop working for 60 days so that performers could be tested. Sharon Mitchell then wrote an op-ed piece in the same paper on 2 May 2004, noting that

> each month we give about 1200 actors a test that can identify HIV as early as 14 days after infection. We also test for chlamydia, gonorrhea and syphilis . . . In 80,000 tests my organization has conducted since 1998, there have only been 14 diagnoses of HIV infection. We're doing an excellent job.

Across the pond, *Arena* magazine in the UK did a piece about the whole fiasco in its August 2004 issue, quoting Jill Kelly as saying, 'Anyone who continues to shoot at this point is a complete idiot,' because while the entire American adult-film industry was shut down for a whole month, certain idiots were indeed still shooting porn. The piece, written by Justin Quirk, ended with a quote from Lara Roxx, sounding very bitter:

> We should think about these issues right now, to change stuff around to make this a safer fuckin' business. It isn't a safe business and I thought it was. I knew double anal [two penises together in the one anus] was dangerous, really, but I was

putting it way back in my mind because I was down in California to make the maximum amount of money, to come back home wealthy. I had plans for the money.

Lara had to borrow the money to return to Montreal. 'After I paid them back for my plane ticket,' she said, 'I spent all my remaining money from that scene. On doctors.'

The poor girl. None of my actual friends ended up infected, though I did know Jessica Dee, but only briefly because we did one movie together – back in 2001, when Stoney Curtis directed both of us in *Fast Times at Deep Crack High, Volume 3*, in which we did a three-way with Mr Marcus, one of my very few interracial sex scenes. Jessica and I appeared together on the box-cover and we shared top billing in the credits. She was so sweet, and was terribly unfortunate to have been one of the girls who did anal cream-pie with Darren James.

Things eventually went back to normal, and the quarantine on performers and the moratorium on production both ended in early May 2004 – a month earlier than expected – after all the suspended talent was repeatedly tested and then cleared to return to work. I broke up with my boyfriend and started shooting scenes with guys again. Still, it was a serious wake-up call.

I have been afraid since then, so I like to see official test results before a scene. If I don't know the guy, I like to see his test and ID, so that I'm sure it's really him. If the test is not from AIM or I can't call for a result, then I won't work with the guy.

Saying that, having a 'current test' sometimes doesn't mean shit, as I've caught things from people whose clean results were 'current' (as, indeed, Darren James's were). You could have fucked someone two days ago and caught something without knowing it. So, I've had sexually transmitted diseases and not recognised the symptoms, or not had any symptoms at all. We should get re-tested if we think anything is wrong at all (such as different smells, different-coloured discharges or abdominal pains).

Every month now, I get stressed out when I go for a test. Although I am now aware of pretty much all the symptoms, having caught chlamydia and gonorrhoea in the past, you never know if you've been infected again or not. If you have shoots booked, then you're screwed, because it takes a week for the medication to work, which also fucks up your insides. I know that I may never be able to have children because of my past STDs (not that I've ever considered becoming a mother – and I've never had a pregnancy scare, thank God – but it's not nice to think you don't have the option), and I get panic attacks all the time, possibly due to some of the medications I've taken.

What pisses me off the most is when I'll only have one or two shoots in a given month and I'll catch something from that one shoot. Off-camera, I use condoms, so I know it's from the shoot. It really sucks big-time

145

when you're only working one or two days and you lose a week of work because of that. This has happened to me more than once, and the reality of what we girls do is that you never know when the next time will be. I mean, why do we do such crazy things, some people outside the industry must ask, to make a living?

These days, most people tend to skip the opening disclaimer that runs just before an adult movie, which reads:

> The sexual situations in the following adult feature are shown for entertainment and informational purposes. We highly recommend that individuals follow the surgeon general's accepted guidelines for safe sex, which are monogamy and/or abstinence, or at a minimum the use of a condom combined with a selective choice of sexual partners. We hope that you find the following feature an enjoyable stimulation to your adult practice of safe sex. Thank you.

I like the 'selective choice of sexual partners' bit – highly ironic, given that we performers seldom get to choose our on-screen partners. We usually work with whoever happens to be cast for that particular movie. There have been times where I deliberately haven't asked who I'm working with because I want to be surprised when I get there and also trust my agent's judgement.

Now, when I do find out ahead of time and then decide not to have sex with that person, that's a different

matter. All of us have a 'wish list' of preferred performers, and sometimes the director will indulge us, but it
doesn't always happen. I used to always choose whom
I worked with but, somewhere along the line, things
changed. It became the directors who would exercise
their choices in terms of guys they liked to use, and
that was that. And as far as 'safe sex' goes, most people
outside the business have no clue what we have to deal
with. At present, every company refuses to shoot with
condoms except for Wicked Pictures, and the general
reasoning behind this is somewhat lame – they claim
that it decreases sales.

I think that's totally absurd. If these guys are right, it
means that the fans are bitching about seeing condoms
in our scenes, which would say to me that they don't
give a fuck about our health – all they care about is
their fantasy, which supposedly gets ruined when we're
shown using condoms! Now, I know this can't be true
of all porn fans, so I think the companies are using it
as an excuse. I even know of one director who actually
said, 'If you don't want to have sex without condoms,
then you shouldn't be a porn star!' – the ultimate in self-
ishness, in my opinion. It's not even written in the law
that we have to get tested every 28 days – that's just a
porn insiders' rule. Things would be a whole lot more
dangerous for us if not for Sharon Mitchell.

If you ask me, the good folks in the United States
government don't care either – they just want to make

sure they earn their share in taxes and that we're not underage or illegal immigrants, hence the 18 USC 2257 Act, which requires the companies to declare on the DVD box-covers that 'all performers depicted in this work were 18 years or older at the time of production'. The whole Traci Lords incident got everyone running scared about using underaged performers, for sure, but there's a whole lot more than meets the eye here. (In case you don't know, back in 1986 porn star Traci Lords was busted for performing as an underaged teenager who'd lied about her age and used fake IDs.) The government basically lets the adult-entertainment industry regulate itself to a degree that isn't always healthy for the people employed, most of whom can barely regulate their own lives. So, it's a case of the blind leading the blind (or rather the blonde leading the blonde, so to speak, not that all of us blondes are stupid).

There are also occupational hazards specifically for the guys in the industry. It can be frustrating for both of us when they have problems keeping it hard, but I understand and will do all I can to help. But some guys just get so intimidated that they can't do it at all! I've had that problem a few times in the past, usually with new guys who think they can make it in the business but get on set and totally lose it.

On one shoot, I arrived to discover it was a boy–girl scene, with a guy I already knew – he was a director himself and used to book me for his own shoots. I knew

he was a big fan of mine and was intimidated by me –
so he was *very* nervous about having sex with me! It
was hilarious. He had to keep leaving the room to get
hard, because he said looking at me was already too
much for him to handle! He smoked some weed, did a
few shots of bourbon and tried to calm himself down,
but nothing would work. Eventually, I gave him some
Xanax and that kind of calmed his nerves. I also had to
keep reassuring him he was okay – I kept telling him
how big his cock was, how good it felt – which helped
a little, except he kept wanting to cum after, like, every
three strokes!

So we had to cut every ten minutes, for him to pull
himself together in the next room for another five
minutes. Then he'd come back hard and we'd start
fucking again. And then he would get the shakes and
he had to go and calm himself down again! We got it
done, eventually, though that went on and on for a few
hours, and all for a 35-minute scene. Poor guy, he may
be permanently traumatised now, with performance-
anxiety issues, all because of me!

It's a huge mind-fuck for a guy, when everyone is
counting on you, waiting for you to perform. Time is
money! And here's where we come to the occupational
hazard. The latest trend for those who prefer not to pop
Viagra pills is caver-jacking (also called CAVR), which
enables a guy to stay erect for long periods by injecting a
liquid into the shaft of his penis. It's definitely not for the

timid, jamming a hypodermic needle into your cock. Most of the guys don't like to admit to it, but everybody knows it goes on. A lot of guys won't admit to taking any sort of drug to help them get hard, but it's pretty obvious when they are rock-hard long before the scene. The guy will then usually stay hard for hours, even after cumming, which must get painful.

Don't get me wrong, there are a lot of male performers who have no trouble getting it hard on their own; it's just that some guys need a little help. The thing that scares me, though, is that by inserting a needle into your cock you leave an open wound – which can be an easy way to contract HIV.

My mantra for all the tricky dilemmas of acting in porn is therefore this: health before wealth.

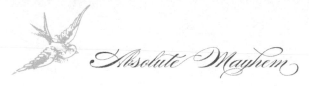

The glamour girl with her new boobs, 2002.

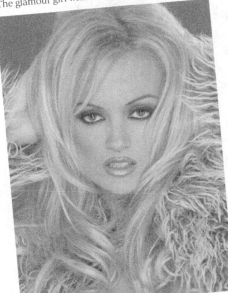

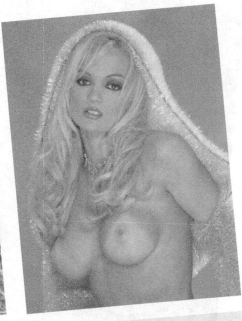

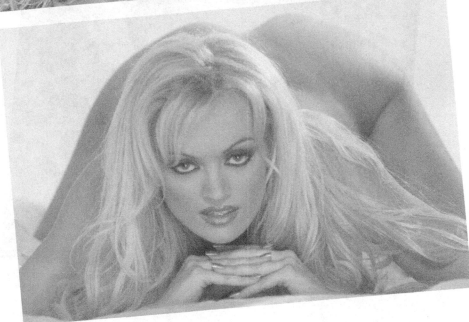

(Photos by Jay Allan)

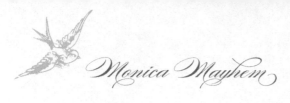

Monica Mayhem

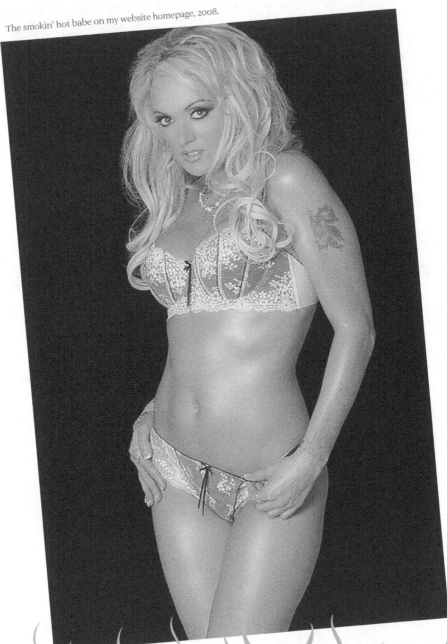

The smokin' hot babe on my website homepage, 2008.

(Photo by Jay Allan)

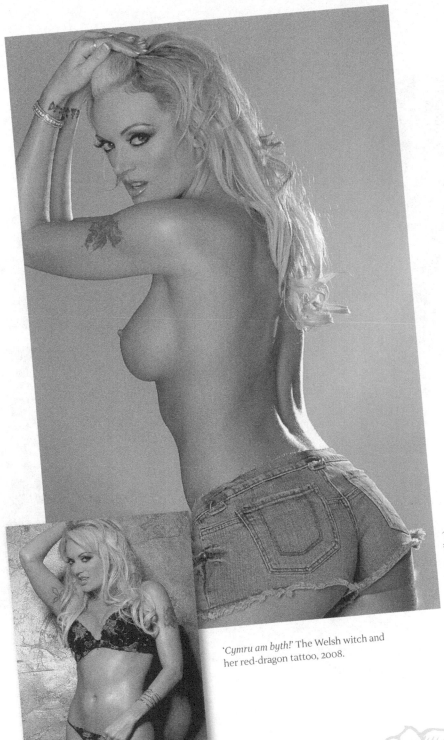

'*Cymru am byth!*' The Welsh witch and her red-dragon tattoo, 2008.

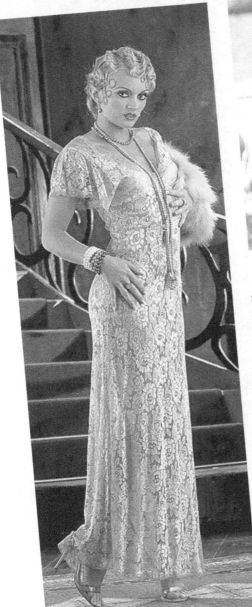

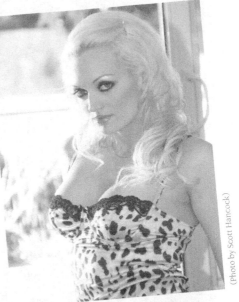

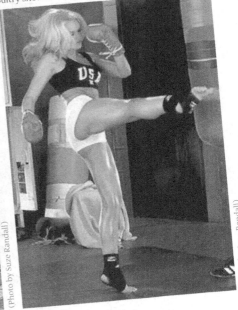

Sultry shot for my website.

Dolled up for a 1920s-inspired shoot.

Kick-boxer extraordinaire!

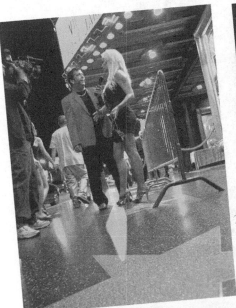

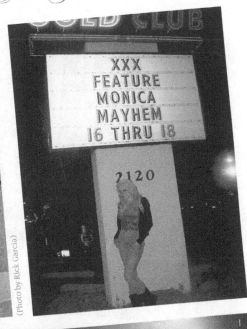

(Photo by Rick Garcia)

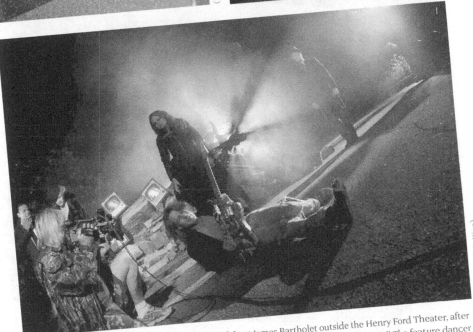

(Photo by Chris King)

(Top left) 'Sure, I love giving head!' With *LA Nitelife* host James Bartholet outside the Henry Ford Theater, after I'd won the 'Golden Throat' Sexopolis award, 2008.   (Top right) 'Brisbane, look at me now!' The feature dancer standing proudly by her marquee, in Albuquerque, New Mexico. (Above) 'Me and my guitar god!' Shooting the 'Rise' video with Eddie Van Halen (guitar) and Barry Wood (camera), for *Sacred Sin*, 2006. My co-star Scott Nails is the masked man on my left.

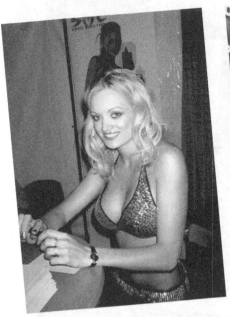
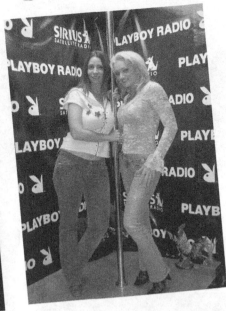
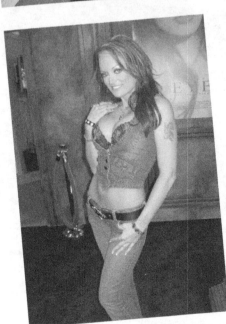
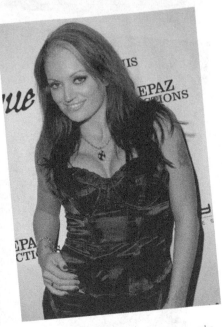

Public (not pubic) appearances. (Clockwise from top left) Signing autographs at the Erotica LA convention, 2003; co-hosting Playboy Radio with porn-legend Christy Canyon, 2008; hot to trot – on the red carpet for the launch of my movie *Skin*, 2006; representing Michael Ninn's Ninn Worx at porn's biggest convention, the AVN Expo in Las Vegas, 2006.

Hangin' with the Hedgehog! With porn-legend Ron Jeremy at The Rainbow on the Sunset Strip, after my gig at the FOXE Awards, 2008.

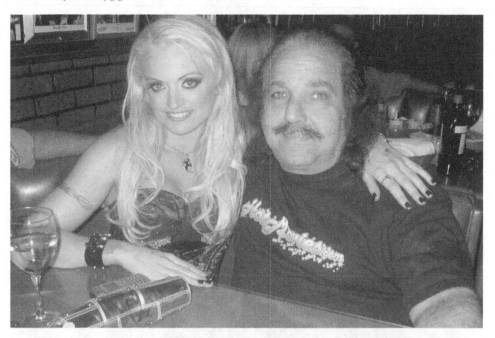

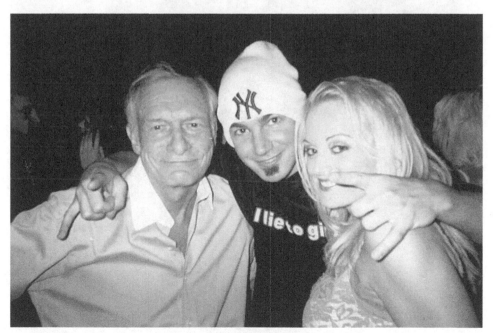

Partyin' at the Playboy Mansion, with Hugh Hefner (left) and Craven Moorehead (now my ex-husband), 2002.

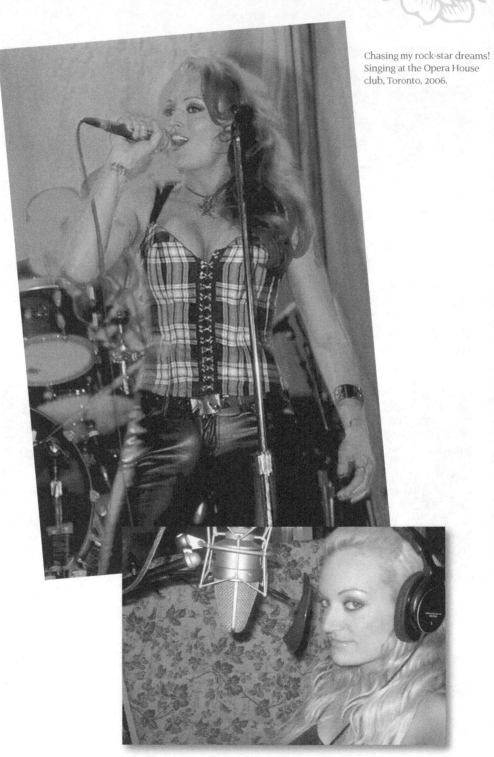

Chasing my rock-star dreams! Singing at the Opera House club, Toronto, 2006.

Recording my song 'Escape' in the studio, Los Angeles, 2008.

Chapter Nine

BEYOND THE
MONEY

So why do some of us girls feel the need to have sex on camera with random guys – and it is a need for some of us, beyond the money, beyond the novelty, beyond the possible lack of alternatives? What's wrong with this picture? Why would you need sex so badly, or need to look good having on-camera sex so badly, that you're willing to be branded as a porn star for the rest of your life and have it colouring everything you do whether you like it or not?

This relates to the 'lost girl' scenario that some writers have noted, the theory that all porn stars are looking for some kind of transcendence, in the same way that young girls who go with older men are seeking out potential father figures or the way nymphomaniacs crave sex as a substitute for love or warmth or shelter. If you ask me, being a porn star is a way of using sex to cauterise our emotional wounds. It is sexual expression as a form of self-actualisation, in order to elevate your own self-worth.

I think that, for a lot of us girls, these sexual acts make us feel worthy of something, in that our audience are getting off on watching us have sex on camera, or even that the guys we are fucking are getting off on fucking us. And it's the knowledge that, somewhere out there, someone is looking at us and admiring us for how beautiful we appear to them and wishing they could have us. It makes us feel wanted for a change, because most of us, in our lives, have never felt wanted or admired or adored. And I, most certainly, have never really felt loved.

I still have issues relating to insecurity, self-esteem and trust, all of which goes back to my messed-up childhood. My enforced freedom at age 14 is very much related to the way I've been drawn into a crazy vortex that has defined my life to date. The freedom to live as I please without catering to an abusive authority figure is very much linked to the freedom to be a sexually expressive person. I began thinking about this because, when you become a famous person, there is such a high price you have to pay, despite the many rewards that come with public recognition, and it's even more so when you're a celebrity in the world of adult entertainment.

Being a porn star is the absolute furthest anyone can go if you're wanting to be famous, that's for sure. How could anyone challenge that? I'm always naked for everyone to see. I do things for a living that most people would consider extreme or outrageous. And it's easy when you get used to it, believe it or not. People expect you to be wild and crazy, which offers a built-in kind of freedom. It's like you're being given permission to enact your private wishes and secret fantasies, for the enjoyment of people who all wish they could do the same but can't. It also helps people like me who spent years being relatively shy and straight-laced. When I got paid to take off my clothes, it was like something in me was finally set free.

Maybe porn is just an easy way for us to obtain those feelings, even if we have to obtain them from strangers, or even if it doesn't mean anything. That's why I appreciate the fan mail I get, and I personally reply to as much of it as I can. As long as it's not stalker mail or hate mail, I'll generally always take the time to sit down and read and reply. For us girls in porn, to even get so much as an email saying how appreciated we are always puts a smile on our faces.

And I do think about how the audience sees me, believe it or not, even if I'm mostly performing for a camera and never see the finished product for months (if ever). This is mostly because I'm out dancing at the clubs too, and I get to size up the crowd. In April 2008, I did a particularly memorable dance gig at a club in Lancaster, California, out by the Mojave Desert. It was actually a bikini bar but nobody told me, so I didn't know there were restrictions on nudity. I promptly took off my top in the first show and the crowd went apeshit.

The management, predictably, were freaking out and worrying they'd get busted by the cops. See, the cops just love to 'randomly' show up at these places, especially when a porn star is in the house (just to make sure we're not doing anything we shouldn't be doing – and, of course, they get to watch a hot performance at the same time!). But nothing happened in the end, except the Pavlovian reaction of the audience. There was definitely a sudden change in their mood, because they were not expecting to see my titties at all. And when I showed them, they all moved closer and started throwing more money and screaming really loud.

In the clubs where I've danced fully nude, I've noticed that the crowd tends to get closer to you and throw down more money because they want to see you up close and personal, fully naked. That's how most guys want to see a porn star, after all. Especially if the girl they've only desired from afar is suddenly right in front of them. When they don't get to see everything, they are somewhat disappointed – I can tell.

So how do we respond to this? By making ourselves look the best we can. We may not want to fuck them in person, but we're going to work at *looking* totally fuckable. That's the whole idea!

On the most basic level, you invest in your body as much as possible. Tanning, for instance, is a major work issue for porn stars. Back in Manly, I had a natural tan from being on the beach every morning (I have an olive complexion and don't burn easily). This was great for when I went clubbing in skimpy clothes, because it made my body look good. Everywhere else, though, I've used tanning beds a lot. When I see myself in pictures with no tan, I think, 'God, I look sick!' But my dad told me recently that I should stop tanning and, as much as I hate to say it, he's right. I have a history of skin cancer in my family and I should watch it. Some of the girls in the industry really overdo it. I'll look at some of them and I can't believe how dark they are for white girls. It makes them look dirty.

I'm not a huge fan of tan lines on myself, but I had to put up with them when I got my breasts done because I couldn't tan my nipples. It was through my nipples that the incisions for my enlargements were made, and I was told that if I subsequently tanned them it would cause deep scarring. My nipples were so sensitive afterwards and it was really bad. For the first two months, even putting a loose top over them would kill me. Their sensitivity is back to normal now, but I still don't like

155

it when they are pinched or bitten. That kind of thing doesn't fucking feel good to everybody, you know? I don't mind my boobs being squeezed or slapped, just not my nipples. I would never do it to a chick, unless she asked me to. There are some guys, though, who like it done to them – they totally get hard when you suck on their nipples!

Aside from my breasts, I've had no other surgery except for porcelain veneers on my teeth. I just wanted a perfect smile. (No one even noticed. My dentist is amazing!) Nose jobs, those I can understand. I hate one side of my face when I'm being photographed, because of a deviated septum from too much cocaine, but I'm actually too scared to have that fixed. But some girls go way too far with their Michael Jackson nose jobs (no disrespect meant to the dead). I've seen lopsided boob jobs, too many facial implants and overly puffed-up lips, too much Botox and 50-kilogram girls getting lipo-suction. By now, I have seen everything that porn has done to the self-image of some girls.

Really, if you just exercise and eat right, and try not to do the cocaine diet, your body will look fine. That's what I tell myself, anyway.

If a new girl comes to me and says she wants boobs like mine, I tell her to make sure she's doing it because she feels inadequate without big boobs, not just for the sake of making it in the business or for what she thinks people want to see. You have to want bigger boobs because you don't feel quite right without them, and because you know it's going to help your self-esteem. The really important thing, however, is to make sure you pick the right surgeon and not just go to someone cheap. As I always say to the new girls, 'Get recommendations from girls with nice boob jobs and pay the price!'

One thing I did think about was a certain phenomenon that occurred not long after my arrival in Los Angeles, when there was a lot of interest in a new medical procedure called 'laser vaginal rejuvenation' in which women were going to these plastic surgeons in Beverly Hills to get their vaginas done. Some of them wanted 'porn-star vaginas' and were willing to pay thousands of dollars to get their nether regions enhanced. We were their role models!

In one sense, I don't think that's strange at all. If women are looking at our pussies on-screen and think that is normal and that is what guys want to see, then why should they not want to be like that? However, what they don't realise is that we are all completely different down there, and guys all have different tastes in how they like a pussy to look. So, really, there is no such thing as a porn-star vagina. Women in general are not bloody perfect, so I'm sorry, guys, but if you don't like how a particular vagina looks then you may be gay! You don't hear us talking about how guys should have surgery to look a certain way, do you? Some girls don't like it when a guy is not circumcised but, to me, as long as they keep it clean and can stay hard, who really cares?

Saying that, my pussy is the part of my body that makes me the most money, after all, and sometimes I do get a little self-conscious about it. It isn't one of those neat and petite ones. After all those years of on-camera sex, I feel as if it's changed in appearance. My labia may not be tiny, but at least I'm still tight down there, even after all that sex. The only downside to that, as I've said, is that big cocks really hurt me. It hurts inside too, and that's why I try not to do too many scenes with hugely hung guys. I'm in pain for days afterwards, especially when I've been fucking for over an hour on some shoots. I get so sore, and that really ruins it for me if I have to shoot again in the next few days.

I do like to keep my pussy clean, and neat and tidy – not because I want to hang it in an art gallery or anything but because I know that some people will be looking at it and analysing it. Beneath a video clip of me for Babestv.com one time, one of the comments said that my pussy was so ugly. That really hurt me. I was devastated. I mean, how cruel, to write something like that! But then I thought that the guy who wrote it was probably so ugly himself that he had to put other people down to make himself feel better. And he had absolutely nothing better to do with his time, and he probably never got laid. And that made me feel a little better about it.

At any rate, when you're working in the adult-film industry, your breasts and other body parts become your lifeline. The sheer reality of this hits you in the face when you're paid that most coveted of compliments – when a company makes a deal with you to produce replicas and you have to get moulds done of your body parts (sometimes just your vaginal and anal regions) for your sex doll. Yep, you get to enjoy getting all that stuff splattered on you and then waiting for it to dry, so that your fans can purchase these products in order to fuck you by proxy. I've been moulded twice now, for my Monica Mayhem love dolls, and it was quite fun, actually.

I have had two sex-toy contracts in my career, first with Topco and then with Pipedream, and the latter were responsible for generating some much-needed buzz for me through their Monica Mayhem 'Saucy Aussie Collection' of sex toys. What I got paid from Pipedream was ten times more than what I got in five years from Topco.

The Pipedream deal was arranged by my manager, Harry Weiss. I'd first connected with Harry around 2005 and was referred to him by Billy Glide, whom I'd worked with many times. Harry got me some of the bigger movies such as *Sacred Sin* and shoots with Wicked Pictures. He's a big Jewish mensch with a good heart, and was very easy to work with. He actually cared about the performers, and he wouldn't get mad if you didn't want to do something. You could talk to him about anything. (As the years went by and more and more agencies were popping up, however, Harry left the business.)

At the time, thanks to Harry, all I had to do was sign on the dotted line. I thought it was a pretty cool idea to call it 'The Saucy Aussie Collection' and I was very honoured to have my own line of toys as a way of embracing the sexy Aussie in me.

When I got my mould done, it must have been a turn-on for the guy that got to do it, since he had his hands all over me. The guy had to do Sean Michaels, the famous black stud, at the same time. I had to help keep Sean hard with my hands while the guy was rubbing plaster all over Sean's cock. Poor Sean couldn't switch off the fact that some guy was rubbing his cock. Of course, I liked it much better than Sean, although the hardest part is where you have to sit still for a whole 20 minutes. It's actually quite a nice, tingly, cold feeling, a bit of a turn-on, and honestly I could have totally masturbated if I didn't have to let the plaster dry!

When my line of toys came out in summer 2007, I signed autographs for trade buyers at the Adult Novelty Expo, which is all about sex toys. I also went to Mexico to do promotional appearances for Pipedream, and it was a real kick. Whereas mainstream models have reached the pinnacle of their careers when they get offered a perfume contract, we porn stars have achieved the same when we get our toy contracts – your own signature line of vibrators, dildos and other stuff.

I got lots of fan mail about the Monica Mayhem love doll from customers who'd bought it and wanted to share their thoughts with me. Now, how about that? They were fantasising about fucking me through using my doll. Some of them told me they thought it wasn't well made because it broke. I wrote back and told them, 'Don't fuck it so hard! It's just a plastic doll!'

At that same toy-trade show, I hung out with other girls who had ranges with Pipedream. For instance, I spent a lot of time with Hannah Harper, just chatting when we weren't too busy. Hannah is English and comes from a small fishing town off the coast of Devon, and she'd entered the industry about a year before me. We were both promoting Pipedream's new product called Sex Water – different flavours of water filled with ingredients such as ginseng and guarana, meant to help enhance your stamina, prolong your pleasure, give you that nice post-orgasmic afterglow and all that kind of good stuff. It tastes a bit like vitamin water, and I guess it's fine if that helps some people. It sometimes takes an event like that to remind me that, yes, we are offering a service that does help people. We bring comfort to those who need sexual stimulation, particularly those with sexual dysfunctions. I see it as an act of compassion and empathy on our part.

The downside of being constantly appreciated sexually, though, is that I am permanently obsessed with my weight. If I see the slightest thing that I think is off, then I will obsess over it. In the past, I have taken diet pills or laxatives a few days before a shoot, because I've felt like I wasn't the perfect weight and the camera adds a few pounds. Most of my fans won't ever point it out, but I'll notice when I am a little overweight. I'm now competing with girls much younger than me and I think my body is much more in shape than most of theirs, because I eat right and I do yoga and exercise. When I was their age, in my early twenties, I could eat what I wanted and never exercise and it kind of sucks now that, after turning 30, I've really got to watch it.

It also doesn't help that, no matter how the porn magazines like to glamorise our industry and make us look as near-perfect as possible, the easy availability of drugs can become a personal problem. There's a very famous porn star who had to stop working at one point because the directors and cameramen and photographers were tired of figuring out how to shoot her so her needle-track marks wouldn't show. She was forced to clean up and eventually made a comeback.

Most of the time, drug use is all about needing to anaesthetise yourself from inner pain. I think that's exactly what I've been doing my whole life. I don't understand why I can't just be sober and be happy with myself. The days when I am sober, I'm so lost and so bored, and I just don't know what to do with myself. I'll try to find a million things to do, but I'm still left feeling lost. I don't ever seem to feel at peace.

It's even harder now, since I've resolved to not smoke weed any more, because that was the one thing that took my mind off everything. I could just escape from reality and be happy and laugh. Now, I find it hard to sleep because my mind is constantly racing about all my problems and about how I am going to fix this and that. My vocal chords love me for it – I gave up weed for music, so I could sing better – but I feel like I also gave up a piece of my soul. I am now finding new ways to achieve inner peace and appreciate everything that I have to be thankful for.

My deviated septum, though, remains a nagging problem. There was one year, 2006, when I was snorting cocaine pretty much every day. Did I have some kind of subliminal death wish? Perhaps. I had been on and off with cocaine since I got into the industry. Prior to that, I had only done it a few times, in Sydney, starting when I was 18, but it was definitely the 'rich man's drug' over there, as it was so expensive. In LA, it's cheap and very easily accessible, so it's very hard to not want to do it when it's around. That is where you really have to use your self-control. And in 2006, I guess I just didn't. I don't know why, exactly, but I know that I was very depressed, so the coke was most probably my way of escaping reality.

Being in the adult-film industry hasn't exactly been healthy for me in this regard. For some people in porn, drugs are accepted as the norm. Although I don't like to be high on set, it's very common for other girls to take drugs while they work. On one shoot that year, one of the other girls whipped out a bag of cocaine and started doing lines between scenes. While I posed for photos, did a ten-minute girl–girl, a ten-minute solo and a ten-minute hand-job, all for three MILF ('mother I'd like to fuck') movies, she was just busting out lines right in front of me! The director didn't know about this, mind you.

I know a lot of girls do speed – which I absolutely hate, especially due to all the friends I've lost to that shit – but I don't even like doing blow and shooting a sex scene. I guess a lot of people get horny doing it, but I never did – it kills my sex drive. Guys totally have it all wrong when they try to lure girls home with coke. They think they are going to get laid, but really the girls just want the drugs.

At some point, I finally realised that I really needed spiritual help. I had to find the path that could bring me comfort and peace – the kind that could erase the emptiness in my life that all the drugs never really filled. And so I began a new life journey and started to find myself again. I made a pact to myself to read up on spiritual healing way more intensively as my New Year's resolution for 2008. The rest of my life was waiting to begin.

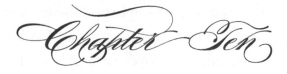

A PERFECT
CIRCLE

*D*o porn stars need spiritual guidance? You bet we do. And more than most people, I would say, given the crazy things we have to deal with. Some of them would do anyone's head in, and sometimes I myself think it's a miracle I'm still sane. So many girls burn out just past their first year, and I could so easily have gone the same route too had it not been for one fateful day back when I was 22, when I chanced to walk into a spiritual bookshop in Woodland Hills called The Psychic Eye.

I realised life's a bitch, so I became a witch.

At this transitional time in my life when I was questioning so many things, being in that bookshop just felt so good and I knew this was it. I bought a bunch of books and supplies, and I studied Wicca for the recommended 'year and a day', a process by which you show your commitment and initiate yourself into the religion. You also need to perform a self-dedication ritual during this time. An important distinction is that I am a solitary Wiccan, and to this day I still practise alone. I don't belong to a coven or even socialise much with other witches, because I just don't trust anyone in LA. In fact, I have only just met another Wiccan girl here: she's the girl who does my facials.

Once I started practising, I found myself with the best, most powerful feeling I'd ever experienced and I felt completely at peace. Ever since I can remember, I'd always felt different. I'd always felt out of place, like I didn't really belong anywhere. I had no religion growing up, but I was always obsessed with medieval times, connecting it with my identification with the Welsh part of me. I do believe that in a past life I have lived in medieval Wales, and that might well be one explanation for my own practise of Wiccan spiritual-ity. (Perhaps I was previously a Welsh witch?) I have always loved books like *The Mists of Avalon* by Marion Zimmer Bradley and anything to do with the story of King Arthur and his fabled Camelot. (Arthur's queen is named Gwenhwyfar, the Welsh spelling of Guinevere.) I collect medieval weaponry and currently own various swords and daggers, even a double-headed mace. (I still need a battleaxe, though. I don't have one of those yet.)

I always get a special charge when I have to play a role that involves dressing up in medieval costumes and riding horses, as occurred when I appeared in an online series called *Whorelore* (www.whorelore.com), originally based on the popular game Warcraft. My friend Dez made the series and I was the first person he thought to call when he was casting the very first episode back in 2006, in which I was the only female character and played opposite an actor named Christian. Dez had chosen me because he knew I could kick-box, fight and do dialogue well, since he needed all three skills as well as the fucking. Christian and I donned our full-on medieval outfits and shot in blistering 46°C heat in Topanga Canyon around the Chatsworth area.

For the first three weeks after it launched, the server kept crashing because the site had something like 500 million hits, and Dez got sent a massive bandwidth bill. He sold a lot of videos and said he had no idea it was going to be so big. He'd started it as a side-project, and now I'm very proud of my place in its success since I was its very first star. Some critics wrote that the series was successful from the start because I was the female lead in the first episode.

I was delighted when Dez brought me back in April 2008 to shoot another episode. The second time around, I did a scene with my ex-boyfriend Barrett Blade and had to ride a Clydesdale horse while dressed in medieval armour – a custom-made steel bra and skirt, plus gloves and helmet and shin guards. I ran the horse around in circles while I was wielding a sword. We shot it out in Ojai, California, in the middle of a forest. I came home all bruised, my hair full of spiderwebs and sticks, and just flopped into bed, hardly able to walk. That was the best scene I shot for *Whorelore* – I really loved it. (At the time of writing, the show is in season two and Dez is hoping to do a 12-episode box-set with extra material.)

Part of being different, or feeling like I was different, meant that I was always trying to be everyone else's psychologist but I would somehow not sort out my own problems. I still do that, but now I realise I was born to use my spiritual gifts to help and to heal others. I am very sensitive to other people's energy. It sucks when it's bad energy because I feel like I have to leave the room immediately and I get panic-stricken. I also tend to read people's thoughts a lot – it's not like I hear them or anything but rather I just tend to say what people are thinking even before they say it. It's like I have a strong sense of the way people are feeling, and I'm very aware of other people's emotions. It's not a Wiccan thing, really, but just the way I am. Being spiritual helps me to notice these things and learn how to deal with them.

This isn't an easy thing to explain, of course. Some people who visit me at home are surprised that I have a Wiccan altar in my bedroom, which is where I pray. Every Wiccan should have an altar and mine happens to be in my bedroom, which is my most intimate personal space. The altar should really be where people aren't going to touch it or even look at it, because it's very personal and not many people understand. The general judgement on us Wiccans is that of the Hollywood stereotype, which is why I usually don't like to say the word 'witch'. Most people are still very ignorant when it comes to understanding the Wiccan religion.

My collection of medieval-type things has led some people to say they think my home has a Gothic vibe. I just hope that people are as open to hearing about Wicca as I am in talking about it, knowing that there are thousands of people around the world who believe in such things.

Basically, Wicca is the 'old religion' – a natural, spiritual practice that has nothing to do with most people's notions of what is 'evil'. In fact, we don't even believe in Satan or Heaven and Hell. There is an afterlife, which some call the Summerland, and there are many gods and goddesses, relating to different things. We believe in 'the threefold law', which is similar to the Indian spiritual idea of karma but with a difference – whatever you do will come back to you but it will happen times three. It could be three times bigger or three times longer, depending on the particular deed in question. Another golden rule is 'And it harm none, do as ye will', which means do what you want as long as you are not hurting anyone.

In Wicca, there are spells and rituals you can do, which involve elements from the earth. Different items relate to different things. Such items include crystals (which can be useful for all kinds of healing), candles, herbs, incense and essential oils. Wicca teaches you to use these spells and rituals to heal and help yourself, as well as others. However, another rule of Wicca is 'to remain silent'. To reveal a spell or ritual you have done will ruin it, so you never reveal anything to anyone, ever.

Before performing a spell or ritual, you should create your sacred space and cast 'a perfect circle', cleansing the area in which you are working and calling all the elements – north is earth, south is fire, east is air, west is water and, finally, there is the ubiquitous element of spirit. These five elements are represented on a pentagram, the five-pointed star with a circle around it, which is a perfect circle (and which is, perhaps not coincidentally, the name of one of my favourite rock groups).

No, guys and girls, the pentagram is not evil! An inverted pentagram is for Satan worshippers (a pentagram drawn upside down to resemble goat's horns) and that unfortunate symbol has been a cause of some anxiety in my life. I used to wear a pentagram chain around my neck but I don't any more, because people who saw it tended to associate it with Satanism. I do wear a pentagram ring, though, on my left index finger, because it's less noticeable. I feel protected with my ring, and it is important to me.

The other problem many people have with Wicca is the whole idea of us casting spells, which they only know from things like the three witches in Shakespeare's *Macbeth*. I personally have never stirred any kind of potion or made a soup in an iron cauldron. It really is regrettable that many people think so badly of us.

A spell, in Wicca, could be considered the equivalent of praying in most other religions, only ours tend to be a little more complex. Sometimes, I'll just sit and pray by my altar, especially when I'm going through a hard time. It makes me feel better. My altar is a wrought-iron and wooden three-tier bookshelf, wrapped in a grape-vine. On it lies a pentagram, lots of candles, a god and a goddess figure, sage (for cleansing negative energy), chalices, a cauldron, boxes full of crystals, oils, herbs, an *athame* (dagger) and many books on Wicca and spells, including my 'Book of Shadows', where I write down all my studies and any spells I have tried.

These days, I don't always cast spells or perform rituals but I do pray and meditate and I sage myself regularly – that always helps when you are feeling negative energy or just not quite yourself. White sage is a cleansing shrub; you burn it and let the smoke float around you.

Oh, and of course I have my broomstick. No, we do *not* fly on them! The sole purpose of the broom is for sweeping away negative energy. Mine is old and traditional, comprising a carved tree-branch handle and black straw. The flying-broomstick thing is just another misconception due to the popular mythologies surrounding witchcraft. Fiona Horne, who is arguably the foremost Wiccan practitioner and educator to come out of Australia, was once asked in an interview if she owned a black cat and a broomstick. She replied that she's allergic to cats but she does keep a broomstick at her front door because the folklore says only people who love you and treat you well will enter your life if you keep it there.

I've never read that myself, and I may try it now, but in my understanding the broomstick is for sweeping away negative energy from any area, especially before a ritual. As for the cat, it neither has to be black nor does it have to be a cat. Seriously. It can be any kind of totem animal. My cat Smokey is grey and white, and is always by my side. He is a little healer. Everyone who crosses his path seems to be enlightened, even if they hate cats or are allergic to them. He has a way about him. Smokey has helped me through many hard times, and a lot of my friends say the same thing. Animals are very spiritual beings and often take after their owners. Smokey is very obedient and sits by my side when I am doing a ritual or praying. I live alone now, but a friend of one of my old flatmates' once asked me if I was a witch – because my cat followed me around everywhere!

I can't blame people for their curiosity, but I will also say that there are people right where I live, in what's supposedly the most open-minded and socially progressive city in the United States, who will baulk or shudder the moment they hear that I'm a real-life witch. Many people will actually say, 'What's that?' or 'Oh, so you're evil!' Or worse, they'll make stupid jokes about it like, 'I'd better be careful around you, then!' It really pisses me off. There's so much ignorance out there. I would like to give these people books to read so they'll understand, but it's a sad fact that most people don't want to know. They live their lives like sheep and just believe what Hollywood or the tabloid press tells them. So I now go by the notion that if people don't take the time to get to know me, they are not worth having in my life.

On the flip side, I have some friends who totally depend on me when they're in need. For instance, an old friend came over to see me last year, someone I hadn't spoken to in about a year. He was going through some really rough times and I was the only person he felt he could turn to for guidance. I believe I helped put his mind at ease. He actually thanked me and I could see that he was happy when he left. You don't need to be Wiccan to do this for someone, of course, but I do believe my own spiritual touch was a great help.

I even have friends who tell people, 'You should hang out with Monica.' They know I will try to help them as I've helped a lot of people overcome a lot of things in their lives. Sadly, most of these people just end up disappearing from my life, without even so much as a thank you. So many people take everything for granted. Well, whatever. At least I feel good about myself for changing a person's life, even if only in a small way or temporarily so.

I know this is true because of what happened with my mother. Despite everything she did to me, I felt sorry for her – so when I heard she was ill I cast a little spell for her health, which had an interesting result. She had been given six months to live but she lived another two and a half years. How much I actually had to do with that I will never know.

As witches, we honour nature and recognise the masculine and feminine principles of divinity. Every day, I thank the gods and goddesses for all that I have and all they are bound to give me. I ask for their strength and guidance to get through each day. I'll also pray for a friend or family member when they're in need.

I find that I can feel the strength of my faith in the simplest of ways sometimes. I love to sit by the ocean and just soak it all in. I feel so energised, particularly if it happens to be raining or if there's a storm. There are some forces of nature that just make me feel so alive. And the full moon is the best time to do any ritual.

That said, it's not an easy spiritual path to explain to the uninitiated if they're not already interested. Wicca, as a pagan religion, should be practised according to the seasonal changes of the land that your physical body is in, so you have to be very attuned to your own physical space. (Fiona Horne rewrote her book *Life's a Witch* for readers in the northern hemisphere after she moved to Los Angeles.) You should only do rituals when the timing is just right, based on whatever you are trying to achieve. You have to get your planets right, your moons right, your days and hours, and it's actually very hard to put it all together in order to do a successful ritual.

I also tend to have psychic dreams from time to time, one of which was about my ex-husband, back when we were still married. I dreamt that he had a hernia. When he came home, I told him and he flipped out. He said I had put a spell on him, because he had just come back from the doctor's, where he'd been told he had a hernia! He really believed I was evil and didn't understand that it was just a dream, a premonition. The funny thing is, after all his believing that witchcraft is evil, he went and got a huge pentagram tattooed on his arm after we got divorced.

Christians love to email me and try to get me to 'accept Jesus' into my life. That drives me crazy, because as a Wiccan I do not judge others for their beliefs. A devout Wiccan would never try to convert anyone to change what he or she believed in. And why on earth would I want to get involved with a group who tortured and killed so many Wiccans during the witch trials back in

175

the sixteenth and seventeenth centuries? What bothers me the most is that one of my best friends became a born-again Christian and almost didn't speak to me any more because I am Wiccan. She was told we were evil, and she didn't understand until she discovered that her 12-year-old daughter is just like me! She didn't understand her daughter either, so she needed me to help her out.

If you ask me, there are all those people who like to say 'This is right' or 'This is wrong' or 'This is the way it should be', when all you really need to know is as long as you believe in yourself and have the universe to guide you, then you will be fine, and for all of your mistakes, you will be forgiven, because no one is perfect. The world is not perfect, and humans are not perfect, and that is what makes us special. That is how we live and learn, and hopefully from our mistakes we become better people. My belief is that if you can remember the basic Wiccan truths, that 'What you do comes back to you threefold' and 'And it harm none, do as ye will', then you should have no problems in life.

I actually have a personal shaman, Troy, who is my spirit guide, and even though he lives in another city in another state, we talk a lot by Instant Messenger. He is one of the few people I can say I trust completely. Troy and I first met on 1 October 2007 on MySpace – who says online social networking isn't useful? We were both looking for spiritual people to talk to. We talk as much as my crazy schedule allows, at least two or three times a week. Most of the time, we chat online, but once in a while he'll call or text me just to check in. He's spiritually pagan, and he believes that Wiccans and pagans are the same – it's just a different name – though he is also in tune with his own Native American ancestry.

Troy's main calling as a shaman is that of a healer, and I know that in the course of the past year and more he has already done a lot to heal me. I feel more grounded now, with his guidance, and he has helped me to refocus my energies and reset my priorities in life. I'm also so relieved that I don't have to keep things inside me all the time and it's so reassuring to have someone to talk to who understands me. He has said that I will do well in the future but things will take time. I need to learn a lot more and train myself, to separate myself from my physical essence and move towards another essence. That's where my music career comes in, and he believes it's a good thing for me. But I have to believe in myself first. 'You are stronger than you even think,' he says.

I have to admit I have a hard time with that, what with all the constant anxiety attacks I get and the kind of self-esteem issues I have. Troy tells me that the most important things I need to focus on are twofold. First, I have to learn to calm down my own mind, because I'm so stressed out and mentally exhausted, and all the things that cause the stress and the exhaustion will not have the same impact on me if I can slow down my mind. The second thing is to cope better with my own eagerness to help out my friends. In this respect, Troy is always advising me about doing 'energy work' – which is his spiritual term for helping others.

'You have the drive and willingness to do such things, but by the same token you have to take precautions and know exactly how to heal, how to balance the energy work,' he has told me. 'You have knowledge of those things, but there is more you need to learn before developing those abilities and using them in helping others.'

It's almost impossible to fully explain the significance of what he has said to me, but I can say for sure that he hit the nail on the head – because those are the two things I have been grappling with my whole life. It's so incredible when you meet someone who can tell you exactly what the very core issues in your life that you need to work on are. Troy has told me that I have a deep hunger and a curious nature about life, that I live for new experiences. We've already had many talks about the people I've associated with and he reinforces my own drive to weed out people from my life who are false friends and don't treat me with respect.

For now, I'm using my spiritual beliefs to help me deal with my daily life. I can do spells and rituals but I definitely don't hex. Real witches who can hex don't ever need to do so. I believe a real witch is a Wiccan, and Wiccan rules say not to hex or do 'black magic', although we are all more than capable of doing so. A long time ago, back when I was new to the craft, I learned my lesson doing a karma spell. I did not know that it was bad to do that, and it did come back to me threefold. The karma spell was basically just a chant saying, 'All the hurt that so-and-so brings upon me shall come back to so-and-so times three.' I thought, 'Hey, as long as this person doesn't keep hurting me, they'll be okay.' But they did keep hurting me, and really bad things kept happening to them.

Finally, they called me out on it and I reversed it, because I felt terrible about it. I guess that shows how powerful Wiccan spells can be if they're done right, though I am restrained by a vow of silence from disclosing any further details as to what exactly transpired between myself and this person. The thing I learned from it, however, is that if you remember to meditate and pray and do rituals, you'll find that Wicca does help you get through hard times. It's only when you stop believing in yourself, when you allow yourself to soak in the negative energy, that you get sucked down into a deadly whirlpool.

One thing I have been asked about regarding my spiritual practice, predictably, is the role of sex. I can't blame people for asking, but they're often disappointed to hear that I have *never* incorporated sex into any Wiccan ritual. However, I am still learning and Fiona Horne has written about practising naked (which we prefer to call 'skyclad') and about how orgasms can be part of Wiccan ritual.

Fiona has even gone as far as saying that powerful energy from her orgasms can propel her spells to fruition, almost like a tantric-sex practice. I myself have never experienced this, nor have I ever included it in my own practice. I mean, I don't disapprove of mastur-bating as part of a Wiccan offering, and I know what Fiona means when she says that 'witchcraft honours sex because in pagan times it ensured the longevity of the tribe'. I would say that we are definitely more free-spirited and open-minded than most other religious groups. My own practice differs from Fiona's in that I don't do rituals naked. Sometimes, I'll wear white for purity. I like to cleanse myself in a bath and then wear clean clothes and sage myself so I'll feel totally cleansed.

However, there is nothing wrong with worshipping when you're skyclad, because many rituals are done that way and that is how we were born and there is nothing sexual about it. It's just natural to be naked, and the gods and goddesses don't look down on you for that. That's the great thing about Wicca – it tells us there's nothing wrong with being who you are and that no one is judging you. How this applies to me is that if I can make a living using my body for other people's pleasure, then there's nothing wrong with that in the eyes of Wiccans. As long as I'm not hurting anyone, I may do as I will. That's the crux of our creed.

On a personal level, I have not engaged in sex with other Wiccans. I have never even had a Wiccan boyfriend, just because I don't really know any. I am a solitary witch and I practise alone. Fiona Horne wrote in one of her books that it was aimed at 'a new breed of eclectic witch emerging now, not tied to a tradition or who hasn't been initiated into an established coven, who perhaps has been drawn to it of their own volition'.

Now, that is so absolutely me. I too am eclectic, which means I believe in all different types of Wicca. I pick and choose from the different traditions. (For those of you who are interested in books on Wicca, I've studied a lot of Silver Ravenwolf and Doreen Virtue, but don't go by my recommendations, because I could be way off as far as what's good for you.) In short, I am solitary, which means I worship without a coven, although that's because I have not yet found one I feel I can belong to or have not trusted the right people to create a coven with.

I only know one other porn star who is interested in these kinds of things, but she is not exactly Wiccan – my friend Noname Jane, who is a 'ceremonial magician'. Ceremonial magic is a practice, not a religion, and it is extremely complex. Its workings are very lengthy. Ceremonial magicians focus highly on correspondences and the correct performance of a ritual, usually called 'high magic'. The ultimate intention is to bring the magician closer to the divine (as compared with 'low magic', which has mere practical purposes and is often equated with witchcraft).

Some girls in my industry claim to be interested in Wicca because they are looking for comfort, but it's really a matter of whether they are spiritual enough and whether they really do feel it. I tell them to study Wicca for a year and a day, and if they can't do that they are clearly not dedicated, so Wicca is not for them. All I can tell them is that Wicca has been good for me. I was born with this gift to be able to spiritually heal or help others, and no matter what happens in my life I will always have my spirit guides to get me through. Although others may call me a freak or not talk to me and judge me for my beliefs, I can't help who I am and what I feel.

Finally, let me say a few things about the impact of Hollywood and pop culture on my spiritual beliefs. We've all seen the TV shows, like *Bewitched* and *Charmed* and *Sabrina, the Teenage Witch*, and movies such as *The Craft* and *Practical Magic*. Fiona Horne said she liked the old *Bewitched* series the best, because she thought 'the incantations were really good' and 'they rhyme and connect with the subconscious effectively'. I think she is right about that, although we can't just wiggle our noses and make something happen. That would be awesome if that's how magic really worked!

In *The Craft* and *Practical Magic*, some things aren't too far from the truth, although you usually don't see results right away. Some of that stuff in those films is actually against Wiccan rules, as you cannot call yourself a true witch if you practise evil.

On the other hand, *Sabrina, the Teenage Witch* is just so far-fetched, and while *Charmed* has some good rituals it is also mostly fantasy. (I can't criticise these shows too heavily, though, because I wrote and starred in that movie called *Witch Coven College*, after all. I don't want to be the pot calling the kettle black!) *The Mists of Avalon*, meanwhile, is one of my favourite movies because it shows the Wiccan side of the King Arthur story. It's somewhat on the mythical side but great fun to watch.

Many people turn to our kind of pagan spirituality for the same reason that Fiona Horne did. She grew up Catholic and decided that Catholicism was, as she put it, 'so sombre and serious, based around mistakes and pain and problems,' whereas Wicca was 'more about having love'. I can relate to that; Wiccans are supposed to lead a life filled with happiness and spiritual healing – of ourselves and others. Wiccans also do not believe in taking money for teaching, which is why we don't have big fancy churches to congregate in. We prefer to use the land and be close to nature. We've never killed anyone in the name of our religion, yet we have been killed so many times – all those witches of yore having being burned at the stake – and still to this day many people do not recognise Wicca as a real religion.

Most people just want to believe what society tells them is right. That is easier for them. It makes it easier to deal with life, and it is easier to follow someone else than go your own way. I believe in what I believe, even though it is actually harder to do so, because I don't believe it should be that easy. You have to do the work or it won't work.

I'm here on this earth, I would say, because I'm proof positive that there is no easy way. Given what I do for a living, which is a double-edged sword, I can testify to that. I've found my spiritual path the hard way, and there's no turning back now. What goes around comes around, as they say. The ephemeral things of this earth have diminished in value, for I've found my own perfect circle.

Chapter Eleven

PORN STAR, ROCK STAR

There are a lot of things you can say about us porn stars, but one thing's for sure – we certainly have a unique job. But it is also a job that makes you very vulnerable, in terms of being left open to criticism and being made fun of. And I don't mean just the nudge-nudge, wink-wink, elbow-in-the-ribs kind of tomfoolery that adolescent boys share when they're discovering sex for the first time.

Not everything that's said about us is good, nor does it have to always be. I can actually understand criticism of this sort, because some girls will go to extreme lengths just for some mainstream publicity and I know that, personally, I wouldn't want to be made to look like a fool just to get more fans and more attention from the media.

One girl did something very risky when she allowed a company that had signed her to a contract to issue a press release saying she'd decided to fuck her fans on camera. She announced that she would select one lucky member of her website a month to shoot a sex scene with her and added, 'It's something that I've dreamt of doing since the very first day in the business. I get all wet and tingly when I think about one of my hardcore fans sliding their hard cock all the way up in me. It's so naughty!'

She was not asking her fans for any money for the sex scene, but they did have to pay to be a member of her website. Once registered, they had to write to her to say why they thought they deserved to win and also what kind of scene they would like to do with her, and she would then pick the winner based on what they wrote. Quite clever, I thought!

The risk I'm talking about is that some people will inevitably call that sort of thing a gimmick that falls into that grey area where porn and prostitution collide. Well, it's grey to those people. Legally, though, porn and prostitution are not the same thing. When there is a camera and a movie involved, it's not prostitution – because the girl is not being paid directly by the guy she's having sex with but by a third party (usually a producer or a production company), so it doesn't count as prostitution.

But in the porn industry there are definitely girls who do 'private' work on the side when the cameras are turned off, and girls who pose for 'private' shoots and get paid by the photographer (for services rendered to him). Personally, I've never gone that far. Back when I was working in the bars and clubs, there were times when I was paid for just being a 'date', which did not involve sex. Sometimes, all I had to do was party with the guy, drink, do some blow, and stay up until he passed out – basically, it was take the money and leave! Some guys were really just lonely and not necessarily looking for sex. They just wanted companionship, so they would pay me to hang out with them.

Even when I was stripping, I never crossed that line. I must have been so naive, because I didn't even realise that the girls around me were doing all sorts of extra-curricular activities. But I wasn't a stripper for long, and when I was feature-dancing I never crossed that line either. I'm sure there are people who think I'm a prostitute, and it sure doesn't help that my name has been included in several escorting websites without my knowledge or permission and I can't do a damn thing about it.

A woman who owned one of these sites, Nici's Girls, got busted but not before she had sold a list of clients and models/celebrities to a mainstream magazine. Truth be told, I get a lot of such offers from various agencies but I don't trust any of them so I never do it. But the damage has already been done – all these agencies have my name up on their sites and I can't do anything to get it taken down unless I pay a lawyer, which wouldn't be worth my while. So everyone thinks I'm hooking too, even though I'm not.

Because of the financial downturn, I'm sure a lot of girls have turned to hooking. I know it would be an easy way to pay off all my loans and bills, but I'm still trying to work the legal way. Am I crazy, not to take the path of least resistance and just go for the money? Maybe so. Time will tell if I'm right.

When I started out in this business, nobody ever told me I'd have to think about stuff like this. After more than eight years of this bizarre lifestyle, I need to find something else to do with my life. I am reminded of it all the time now, every time a shoot gets cancelled because some silly girl flaked out and didn't show up, or whenever some amateur pornographer who thinks he's a director tries to make a movie. There have been dozens of such scenarios, and the list seems endless.

Mine is a career where you're dealing with extreme behaviour of all sorts, all the time. The whole issue of hate mail is a good example. Bluntly put, there are some people out there who have too much time on their hands and choose to inflict their own all-too-obvious insecurities on other people. Porn stars, of course, are an easy target.

Back when I was brand new in the adult-film business, I did my very first interracial sex scene. One very disturbed individual chose to express himself somewhat negatively. He sent me a letter that clearly reflected all the wit and sophistication of the KKK, of which I can only presume he was himself a member.

It read like this:

> How dare you go and fuck that nigga with that turd colored cock and that poisonous semen?! If I were your father or brother, I would beat the living hell out of you! You make me sick, you fucking white trash whore!

Pretty eloquent, huh? I wonder whether he did remedial English in high school. Things haven't improved much in eight years. Recently, another guy sent me some nasty, judgemental comments about porn stars. I promptly rewarded his trouble by publishing his rant on my blog and cited his name, since he had so kindly left his MySpace address. The 36-year-old lug from Louisiana had written to tell me:

> You are a hooker-porn star. Why don't you go suck some cock to get rid of your money problems? Isn't that what you porn stars do when you are short on money? I have fucked seven porn stars and your kind are easy to figure out. Go turn a trick, you trick.

Wow, I thought, what a vocabulary this boy must have, to make such exceptional use of the English language!

I wonder if those seven girls he claims to have slept with were truly 'easy to figure out'. What makes him an authority on porn-star psychology? Seriously, don't some people have better things to do? I posted on my blog a direct retort to him:

> You don't fucking know me, so quit being so quick to judge! I am a good person, with a big heart, and the people closest to me know this.

That's the best anyone can do when faced with bigots like these.

There will always be men out there looking for ways to put women down, and when a woman is so obviously open about her sexuality these guys act like sharks sniffing blood. I think a woman who allows herself to be a sex object should be put on a pedestal, because sexual objectification is a form of worship, like they did in the early pagan religions. But how can you explain that to these guys?

Jessica Drake, who starred with me in a hilarious movie called *Hi-Infidelity*, once gave an interview in which she talked about this in a way that I can very much identify with. 'I am a sex worker,' she said. 'I got into this business to do that, so that people could see me have sex on camera, for the attention. I want it. Everybody look at me – me, me, me! And I like the fact that I inspire people. I realise that I provide a fantasy and I'm fine with that. I want to be everybody's fantasy.'

I guess I, too, am a sex worker and it does come down to wanting attention. It really is nice to have fans and to have people appreciate you for being brave enough to display the sexual side of yourself – not too many people you meet on a daily basis can claim to be this way – and so, to be seen as someone who represents a 'good fuck' can actually be a wonderful thing. I like being thought of as someone who can provide pleasure.

I often do live chats for my website, and most of the time these sessions are done from my bedroom, so I can get naked in a comfortable place. I really want whoever's watching me to get off on enjoying what they see. I like the thrill of the real-time interaction – they can watch me talk dirty and pleasure myself, while they do the same.

I don't expect everyone watching to be jerking off to me, because sometimes these guys just want some time to talk to me, and it's hard when so many other guys are asking me to do certain things rather than making small talk. But when I see a guy on my website's chat room going crazy as he brings himself to orgasm, I get really excited and I'm like, 'Yay! Done my job!' As a porn star, that's what you're supposed to do. I took to this like a duck to water, right from day one.

I really believe that porn has an important social function. The primary reason most people are drawn to it, and to its stars, is the sense of experiencing the 'forbidden', so we are actually providing a useful and beneficial public service by helping guys (and girls) to attain sexual pleasure and achieve sexual release without hurting anyone. I believe this, absolutely, with all my heart.

I feel that without porn, there would be so many more sexual predators out on the streets. We are fulfilling a lot of fantasies that most guys or girls don't otherwise get to experience. A lot of my fans thank me for saving their marriages, and that makes me feel good. I'm also happy that a lot of guys who don't get laid as often as they'd like to are dependent on me (and my scenes) to get off. And, as sick as it sounds, all those paedophiles out there are getting a good dose of what they'd like to see and therefore are hopefully staying at home watching fake young girls on their screens rather than actually preying on minors.

Here's what I'd say to the conservative folks who like to hurl their narrow-minded criticisms at us: 'Whatever other fetishes these people have, don't you think it's better they get to watch it on DVD or on the internet, rather than trying to make their fantasies come true by harming innocent women?' When you look at it that way, we are really saving a lot of lives and helping a lot of people with their own sex lives. Without porn stars, there would be a lot of sexual chaos in the world. So much more sexual frustration would be taken out on innocent victims.

Porn Star, Rock Star

What the people who like to criticise us don't see are the inner workings of an entire industry and the dynamics that make it turn, including the money and deals that grease the wheels. We porn stars are dependent on other people for our living – agents, managers, publicists and also the writers and editors of the magazines – so by lambasting us these people are also hurting them.

They also don't see that we have to work with the press, which means you won't last long if you're just some blonde bimbo. This is a tough ball game, because it seems like you have to kiss ass to a lot of editors, which I was never one to do. I'm always friendly and courteous to writers, but I'm not an ass kisser. In general, you really have to watch what you say, because some people will either twist your words or, worse, record everything word for word when you didn't mean to say something the way it came out. That's always difficult, and you just need to think hard before answering some questions. It never gets any easier dealing with people in this business. Instead, you just get more and more used to it.

I also think this industry gets a bad reputation because some of the girls who give interviews to the press are not exactly the brightest light bulbs, so people think we're all ditzy or stupid. They don't realise that it takes some smarts to survive in a business where your success often depends on how well you can find people whom you can trust and rely on. It isn't easy at all, and you have to manage not to burn out from the sheer fatigue of dealing with the whole charade.

I trust my own intuition and I think I always seem to know what is going to be good for my future, even if it's not what normal people would consider a good career move. I feel quite sure I now know a lot more about sex than most people, thanks to all the experimentation I've done in the name of cinematic and photographic art.

And now, for the sake of many of my fans who are dying to know about my own approach to sex, I'd like to set the record straight. The question about sex that seems to intrigue most people is this: do male porn stars turn me on, or are they just 'prop dicks' to me?

Some male performers still turn me on, especially when it's someone I haven't worked with for a while, unless they've really let themselves go with their appearance – that is *such* a turn-off to me. I like a guy who takes care of himself the way I do, but not too much, just enough to look healthy and toned, rather than fat, sloppy and hairy. However, if they have that same sexual appetite they used to have, that can make up for a bit of slackness.

I like passion, and I hate it when guys act like they are just there to fuck you and get paid. I'm sure that if you ask the guys how they feel about the girls they have to work with, they'll all say pretty much the same thing. It's so much more fun when they are really turned on by me and when they make me feel like they are there for me and not just for the pay cheque.

Now, I have to add the obvious – some guys automatically assume that porn stars will fuck anything, just because of what we do for a living. These are the guys who will try to make passes at us at parties or try to cop a feel or get a free grope of any of our body parts in public. Seriously, that's not very smart on their part. When you stop to think about it, it's a really dumb assumption. If we fuck for a living and get paid to do that, why would we want to fuck any random guy that comes up?

While it is true that some girls in this business will fuck just about anyone, those are the very girls any normal guy should avoid – for no other reason than the fact that those girls are always the ones who end up bringing sexually transmitted diseases into our circle, because they're so reckless and don't use condoms.

Getting accosted is one of those things that becomes an occupational hazard when you meet men at parties. I've had to change my phone number numerous times because of obsessed guys or because of people getting my phone number from people I hardly know who then call me up and try to ask me out. It's a pretty common practice for girls in porn to change their mobile-phone numbers every six months or so to avoid potential stalkers.

In general, the best thing to do if you're a porn star is to use a separate email address from your regular email and never give out your phone number unless you want someone to call. There's no easy way to handle these kinds of situations, and I find I just have to compartmentalise my life. Yes, it will suck if, some day, no guys will want to try hitting on me but right now I just get creeped out when I see how desperate some guys are. They'll see a porn star and drool like dogs on heat.

However, those guys usually make it easier for me to spot the guys I do want to fuck – they're usually the quiet ones who don't make it so obvious that they're looking to get laid. Now that, to me, is way more of a turn-on than some cocky bastard who thinks you're there for the taking. Some guys do get nasty when you turn them down, though, and they'll turn on you by saying things like, 'You're just a fucking whore anyway!' They're just hurt that I've rejected them, so I've learned to ignore those kinds of insults.

The other problem that arises, particularly in my case, is when I'm networking and talking business with guys who may be able to help me in some way or other. Sometimes, it's not easy to tell when they're serious about working with me on something and when they're just trying to date me. I've had crazy situations where I've regretted giving my phone number to one of these types, because they'll then keep calling or texting me to go out with them. I end up not taking those calls or screening my calls – because once you return their call, there'll be no end to it. They'll keep bugging you to 'hang out' or 'meet for dinner'. This tends to happen quite often to me because I'm trying to get a rock band together and some music-business types can be so obnoxious.

My own love life hasn't been rosy. It's difficult maintaining a normal personal life, even if you socialise within your own work circle, like a lot of mainstream Hollywood actors do. I've only actually dated one other fully-fledged porn star and that didn't work too well at all. I think it is partly to do with my own inability to open up quickly. It usually takes me a good six months to really give in and let go of my own emotions. Guys also get very insecure with me, because I don't ever tell them how I feel. I'm always afraid of falling in love and then being left alone, which seems to be a recurring pattern in my life. So I try to hold back.

Anyway, I don't like to date within the porn industry any more because there's just too much drama – people are always trying to hurt you by telling you things about your man that you don't want to hear, especially right before you're starting to shoot a scene, which really messes up your mind.

Now, I keep things strictly on a professional level, so that when I go to work I have no emotional attachments to anyone I work with. You have to learn to separate love and sex in this business (and the operative word there is 'learn') because a lot of people confuse the two. You can fall in love so easily just by having sex with someone. But they are two totally separate things. You can fall in love with someone without having sex with them. I do think, however, that good sex is key in a relationship. If you don't have good sex, you're doomed to fail.

As for myself, I think I'm just scared of falling in love and being hurt, and I get very depressed about this. Again, it stems from my childhood issues of feeling abandoned and neglected, so I put my guard up with every guy I meet. I also know that my single biggest problem is that I get bored easily. I've had so-called relationships where I've dated guys and we didn't last three days together.

I don't fully know why it seems so hard for me – I see all these happy couples in the business and I think I'm very sincere. Maybe I need to pick stronger men, who are more emotionally secure. All the guys I meet want to be famous too; they want to be the one in the spotlight. I'm holding out for the right guy still, but as of this writing he's nowhere in sight. (As a tip, if you've got tattoos, piercings and a shaved head, that will tend to boost your chances.)

As far as what I like in bed, well, I've had sex with guys who can cum more than once or who can hold it in, but, to me, when they hold it in too long it seems to take them forever when I do want them to cum. And that makes me feel inadequate. I like it when the guy is so turned on that he wants to cum right away. Feeling guys cumming is a huge turn-on for me, as long as it's not within seconds of fucking me, or from just getting a blow job. I'm really not a fan of 'marathon' sex. I know a lot of guys think they're really good for being able to have sex for long periods of time.

But, in reality, it gets old after a while, and girls get sore down there.

Not only that, as I've mentioned earlier I have a hard time cumming from just penetration, unless I'm in love with the guy or he is just really good at staying hard inside me while I grind on him long enough for me to bring myself off. I do get pleasure from penetration; it's just very hard for me to achieve orgasm this way. So, realistically, long sessions of fucking do nothing for me. I would rather a guy came quickly than have him trying for hours to please me. But hey, if we were dating and still getting to know each other, I'd say, 'Don't give up!' When I am comfortable with a guy, the sex is different. It's just those few awkward times in the beginning that go on too long, where we're not connecting spiritually and sexually, in which you might just become one of my 'once every couple of months' type of guy. (Oh yes, I do have those.)

I don't tend to like it when guys get too attached to me, though. I think I have some kind of attention-deficit disorder, even when it involves sex! Poor guys – I have to set them free. I think that makes me a really great porn star, since having numerous partners is never a problem for me – I like the freshness and the variety, and I'm never one to complain when a hot new guy or girl comes my way.

But if I am *seriously* dating someone, then the poor guy just doesn't have a chance. Once I'm stuck on a guy, I can't even look at someone else. That's the old-fashioned, romantic side of me, I guess, which isn't always a good thing. Maybe that's why I don't show that side of myself very often, and why people tell me how cold I can be.

Often, I cringe when people show me genuine affection. I never knew how to say those three deceptively simple words, 'I love you', and I still don't. It's so hard when you're not used to being loved or being hugged.

So, if you're a guy dating me, be prepared to be pushed aside, especially at a red-carpet event or anywhere where there are a lot of fans. You'll mostly have to stand in the background and wait, because you're going to have people grabbing me and pushing you aside, even if it's just going out in clubs in Hollywood. That's how it's been with every guy I've dated since becoming a porn star. And that's another reason why it's been so difficult for me to have a relationship, because most guys are so insecure. They don't believe that I'm actually faithful and loyal. They think I'm after every guy or something, and they don't believe I can love them.

What usually happens is they either just leave me or they cheat on me, thinking I'm doing it to them when really that's just the way my career goes, since I'm always having sex with other people.

Seriously, guys, try asking me out if you want to date me and then remember this: every time I'm sucking on some guy's cock and letting him spew his sperm all over my face, I do it because that's what I do for work. Think you can handle that? Yeah, right.

I've had my heart broken more than once this way, the most recent case being over the rock star I was seeing on and off for a few years. He lived in Montreal and was on tour most of the time, but we had a very strong connection. For so many reasons, he was the love of my life, my soulmate, but so many things kept messing it up – and a lot of that was to do with me being in porn. I'm not one to give up that easily, but when things become too painful it's easier just to walk away. I think now that our relationship is, regrettably, finally over.

A graphologist who analysed my handwriting said some interesting things about me that I thought were quite accurate. She told me in her emailed analysis that my handwriting belongs to a person who is

ambitious, strong, and energetic, but not grounded. Someone who has plenty of drive, like a sense of mission, and who also has a very clear sense of what money is worth but somehow isn't grounded – meaning that you tend to kind of spacc out a bit. You used to do that a lot as a child, more than as a teenager, and you had a childhood that was probably neglectful. From a young age, you created a sort of bubble for yourself and lived in this private space, like another universe. You used to live in a bubble and you used to dream and kind of space out.

She also said that I am a very direct person who doesn't hide behind mannerisms, and that I have good observation skills and am good with small details, though I sometimes lose track of the bigger picture. I was stunned when I got that analysis, as it was all based solely on my handwriting. I did live in a private bubble when I was a kid, and, to some extent, I find myself still doing that. The porn industry is a microcosm of really unique and unusual proportions and we're all living out little dreams through it.

And as for small details and the bigger picture? Well, my memory for detail is quite astonishing. I can remember obscure things about many movies I did and even name the locations of certain shoots. There were some still shoots that I did with Robbye Bentley in Simi Valley, Southern California, back in 2001, for instance, that I remember like it was yesterday. I can also look at some of my old layouts and name the photographers right away – Jay Allan, Hank Londoner and Scott St James, in particular – and I can talk about strange or funny things that happened there with blinding detail.

For example, there are some photos where the guy's face isn't even in it but I know who he is – because I can recognise his cock! There's one shot I really love, where I'm on all fours looking lewdly at the camera while the guy is spraying his sperm on my lower back, and only his hand clutching his dripping cock can be seen. But I recall not only who he was but also what else he did: right after that, he leaned over and slurped up his own cum off my back! That was pretty nasty. But then again, at least it was his jizz and not some other guy's! (Although, as I later found out, he likes to swing both ways.)

On the live internet show that I co-host every week (*Smell My Finger*, on Rude TV), I recently played an entire scene from one of my movies, *MILF-O-Maniacs 2*, directed by Mark Stone for Wicked Pictures, shot in November 2007, and I gave the audience an impromptu running commentary, as if I was doing a voice-over commentary for a DVD 'Bonus Features' section. The scene featured me and Alex Sanders, and just watching myself hold a certain position immediately brought back what it was like when I was there. I could recall the pain in my legs when Alex was fucking me doggie-style as I kept one leg up on a narrow table that was more like just a ledge. And when we did reverse-cowgirl, with me standing over Alex but facing the camera, so you could clearly see Alex's cock sliding in and out of my vagina from a low angle, I spontaneously said, 'Now, that's really good for cardio and it's a great leg workout too!' (Girls, are you paying attention? That's what you can do the next time you're too lazy to hit the gym!)

I also recall doing one of my favourite films, *Hysteria*, and how I wanted to kill the director, Darren Kaye, for making me masturbate throughout *every* scene in that movie. I was so raw after half a day of shooting, and I had to do it for two whole days. Masturbating was his fetish, though, and we became good friends from that movie and I forgave him. But I vowed never to do that again. I do love to masturbate, but not to that extent – I mean, that was over eight hours per day, which was ridiculous. I love to do it in private, and during sex, and on those live webcams – I like to watch guys jerk off while I masturbate. If they've got their webcam trained on their face, I ask them to move it down to their cock. I especially love it in real life: if they can't make me cum, then I make them watch while I make myself cum.

When it comes to moving beyond the details and sizing up the big picture, I'm a different story. The graphologist said that I tend to suffer from sudden bouts of anxiety and I can be aggressive when I'm put in charge of people – she says I shouldn't ever try to run a company because I get too stressed out and I agonise too much whenever I make a mistake. She added that despite what I do for a living, I am actually a very private person, which I think is true. I have a very strong sense of my own privacy.

She also said that I kind of 'swing between needing people and not needing people, and also between needing to please people and not needing to please people'. That's not atypical of many of us who work in entertainment. I am often very conflicted about my social relationships and I find myself second-guessing whether certain people can be trusted. Los Angeles is a city where you have to learn very quickly who you can trust or else you'll waste precious time dealing with the wrong people. As one famous movie producer, Lynda

Obst, once said about working in Hollywood, 'Nobody has friends, we all only have alliances.' This is almost impossible to explain to anyone who hasn't lived and worked in LA, a city that's actually much less laid-back than its legend claims.

I think, ultimately, it's that peculiar trait of my personality that makes me realise I'm not meant to stay in this business much longer. The thought of leaving porn crosses my mind every now and then. I do sometimes think, though, that since I do take care of myself and my body, and everyone keeps telling me that I look better than I've ever looked, it means I still have a few more good years left. And, if the MILF craze continues, I'll have plenty of years of work left.

In the past few years, any girl who's 25 or older qualifies as a bona fide MILF, and you can film her acting like she's a hot, sexy mother who'll want to fuck anyone behind her husband's back. (There's an even sillier sub-genre called GILF – yes, grannies – which I think is just ridiculous.)

But every girl in this business has a shelf life and the parts definitely get fewer and further between once you've hit your 30s. Because of the constant influx of new girls, the agents and managers and producers want fresh faces and younger girls all the time. That's partly why my music is starting to become more and more important to me. I've been writing a lot of songs over the past two years, with the aim of releasing my first album some time in 2010. That's my immediate goal, anyway, even though some people think I'm crazy.

Admittedly, this isn't the first time I've set my mind to becoming a rock star – far from it. Back in 2004, I did an interview with *Rock Confidential Online*. The headline of the story read, 'Monica Mayhem: Hot Pornstar on her Way to Being Hot Rockstar'. That was after they'd heard my demo song 'Take This Away', which I had written with a friend (who shall go unnamed here), who had previously written for the band Korn.

It was a very hardcore song, and my friend even screamed during the chorus to give it that extra edge. We wrote a lot of great songs together, but all unfinished – because, as usual, he wanted more than just to make music with me. All I wanted was to work together, and we could have gone so far with the music we had created, but he wouldn't even let me keep any of the ideas. I tried working with other musicians after that, but the music just never came out the way I wanted it to.

I spent a lot of money recording songs, paying musicians to play and having the songs mastered. But I didn't like any of them. I also had many meetings with managers and people in the music industry, all of which (yes, as usual) were talking to me because they were trying to fuck me. Or, worse, were telling me that I had to sleep with the chief executives of certain record labels in order for me to get a deal – which, obviously, I did not do. I didn't believe for a minute that they would give me a deal just like that.

It wasn't until 2006 that I finally found that successful writing chemistry again. This time, it was with a great guitarist, Cordell Crockett, formerly with the band Ugly Kid Joe. I met Cordell through a woman I'll call Jane, a friend of my tattoo-artist friend Maxx. Jane was a drummer and introduced me to Cordell because she thought we might be able to write some music together. And she was right.

We got right to it and wrote some awesome songs. I then met a producer who was dating one of my flatmates at the time, and I played him some of our demo songs. He said, 'You've got potential here. If you can put together an all-girl metal band, I'll set up a showcase for the labels.'

And that's exactly what I did. First, there was Jane, who was such a great drummer. However, she sometimes got distracted – by doing lines of coke in the middle of a song during practice! (Admittedly, I was similarly distracted too, at times.) Then, Jane introduced me to another girl, who was a bass player and who was, to put it mildly, a wee bit crazy. (I won't name her here.) This girl was all over the place; she would jump from one thing to another and never finished a whole song during practice. We also had Cordell's friend Deralyn, who became our guitarist.

She was technically great on the guitar, but jamming (in order to come up with song ideas, which is how I prefer to work) really wasn't her thing.

And the drama began. Most of our practices consisted of drinking beer and doing blow. (For me and Jane, anyway.) However, our crazy bassist was shooting up speed, and after I found out I told Jane she needed to tell her that I didn't want to be associated with someone who did that. Because, to me, that was crossing the line. That girl was just a loose cannon ready to explode. When Jane told her, she lost it. She said she was going to come after me and shoot me in the head! (See? That's why I didn't want to mention her name!)

To cut a long story short, there were all sorts of dramas with this all-girl band, including changes of personnel that were just as unsuccessful and dramatic as the previous line-ups had been, and the whole thing eventually fell apart.

Fortunately, throughout all this Cordell and I never stopped writing together. I got invited to play a gig in Las Vegas in 2007, so Cordell brought in his friend Harley to play drums. He was a really awesome drummer. Cordell would play the riff and Harley would get the drum parts right away. We couldn't find a bass player in time for the gig, but we did it anyway by splitting the signal on stage so that the guitar would also produce the bass line. (It was very complicated, and I really don't know how they did that!) We went by the name of Sweet Avenge and did an awesome show in front of a bunch of bikers, who even cheered on my love song 'Never Again'.

I then played our demo songs to an exec at Roadrunner Records, the label behind heavy-music bands like Dream Theater, Megadeth and Slipknot, and he said that we needed live drums (true, because they were computerised) and more lead guitar. I honestly didn't think we were hardcore enough for that label, but the music exec said to come back when I had the songs recorded in a studio, and this got me feeling all pumped up.

However, this band was also doomed. Perhaps we were not meant to be. It started with Cordell and Harley getting into a big fight one night. From that juncture, Cordell and I continued to work together, but Harley was out.

We managed to find two new musicians just in time for another Sweet Avenge gig, at the FOXE Awards in 2008. There was Sara, a great make-up artist whom I'd worked with on Playboy TV and who turned out to be a great bass player too, and her boyfriend, Charles, who was an amazing drummer. By then, Cordell and I had written and recorded eight songs together – all, in my own estimation, great songs – but we were only able to do three songs at the gig, as we really didn't have enough time to get the band together to practise doing any more than that because of all our clashing schedules.

I also landed us a gig performing in a music video for my 2008 movie *Rockstar Pornstar*. This was a porn film written just for me, as everyone in this business calls me the Rockstar Pornstar! It was basically a mockumentary about my 'amazing' double life, including interviews with the band, me fucking groupies, groupies fucking each other, and, of course, the music video.

The only thing was, Cordell didn't have ID, and you have to show valid ID in California to appear in a porn flick, regardless of whether or not you are performing music or sex or just playing a janitor. In the end, we had to use Charles's friend Cyrus in the video. Cordell was not happy about this, of course, but there was nothing I could do about it.

Cordell was having some personal problems around this time, which weren't getting resolved. And my band members wanted nothing to do with him, so again I'd lost all of my musicians – eventually including Cordell himself. He went away to Hawaii for a while and came back with a new outlook on life. However, he is now involved with another female musician and is currently working on a project with her.

This leaves me with all these unfinished songs and a ton of melodies I've written that are just waiting for a musician of his calibre to come and put music to. If I could do it on my own, I would, but I'm not good enough on guitar – not good enough, I would say, to write music on my own at the level that I aspire to.

So here I am once again, trying to find that next musician to share that great writing chemistry with. Cordell has assured me that he still wants us to work together, but he just needs to sort a few things out first. I can't wait forever, so I'm on the hunt right now for new musicians to work with. Maybe, I'm now thinking, I'll save myself a lot of headaches and just hire musicians.

The music business, everyone tells me, is even more twisted than the porn business. Yes, I know, it's full of conniving tricksters and sleazy scumbags. Dyanna Lauren, who was a singer before she became a porn star, once explained her career change this way: 'I decided that if I was going to get screwed, I would at least get paid for it.' But I'm going to give it my best shot.

I've already had meetings where I know that these guys know I'm a porn star trying to get a record deal, so at first they're all thinking, 'Oh, whatever.' Then they actually hear my music and my voice and they're shocked. It's kind of a nice surprise for them, and I'm treated way more respectfully after that. You can't bag on someone if they actually have talent.

There have been porn girls in the past who have tried to break into the music industry but probably didn't have talent, so I naturally get stereotyped. And then there have been those who had talent and didn't make it anyway. Heather Hunter scored a deal with

Island Records when she was a Vivid Girl but her album bombed. Lorraine Lewis, who was a stripper, had a great band called Femme Fatale and managed to release one album on MCA Records, and that stiffed too. Traci Lords made a great album, *1000 Fires*, but it just didn't work beyond the electronic-dance/trance niche market.

I wonder if I'm going to be one of those casualties in today's music wars. Usually, I try not to tell people I'm a porn star, just to see how they react to my music first. I do come from the country that produced Chrissy Amphlett, after all, so I hope there will always be a place for sexy Aussie sirens who can rock.

If nothing else, as a singer I'll be able to become the object of men's fantasies in a different context. I have no problem with that at all. The radical feminists will hate me for saying this, of course, but I think it's a huge compliment to a woman if you think of her as attractive enough to be fuckable. That's one of the key reasons why I became a porn star in the first place. It was such a relief for me, to be allowed to express this in an open way rather than by stealth and subterfuge – which is what you do when you work in financial markets and are forced to be a secret slut in a corporate uniform. I did that for six long years.

Of course, becoming a porn star has brought its own share of problems unique to the profession, but that applies to any line of work. I can say, with a clear conscience, that I don't regret one bit what I chose to do after I left Salomon Smith Barney in London, and not a lot of people could say the same about their career path.

Meantime, I'm going to keep on celebrating and enjoying my own sexuality. That's kind of a weird thing to say at this particular time, when the industry is in a serious recession. A lot of girls have given up and are trying to get normal jobs. A girl who's actively working in the industry right now will be doing maybe three scenes per month, while a lot of girls aren't even getting one scene a month and have to supplement their income with escort work.

And so, I have also found myself auditioning for mainstream movies, with mixed results. In late 2007, I made a fantastic breakthrough when I was cast in a small role in a mainstream movie. And not just any mainstream movie: this was *Sex and the City*. When I auditioned for it, the casting directors took a Polaroid of me, along with several other blonde girls, and then they came back and told me and a couple of other girls to wait. They called me in first, and said, 'You were the director's favourite, but can you just show us that you can fake having sex?'

I said, 'How? Where? Right here on this chair, by myself?'

One of the casting directors replied, 'Yeah, or whatever you're more comfortable with.'

So I just rode the chair. I rode it like I was having sex, reverse-cowgirl style. Bucked my hips, rocked my thighs, and just let it rip.

When I finished, they asked if I was available on the days they wanted, and once they'd called Harry Weiss to confirm, that was that. My first-ever part in a mainstream Hollywood movie, and it was so much easier than I'd imagined! It was a small part, but all I had to do was be myself, both in terms of getting the role and then doing the real work. (Whose idea was that to hire a real porn star to play 'Dante's Lover', which was how I was finally credited? Not that I'm complaining.)

When I arrived on the set, all I could see were about 20 trailers. Kind of confused about where to go, I asked a crew guy, 'This is *Sex and the City*, right?' I told him I was shooting and he directed me to the production manager, who took me to my own trailer. It was small, with a bed, table and bathroom, but it had my name on the front so I felt a little special. I had a nice big meal and then sat around waiting to be called for my scene. I sipped hot chamomile tea, as it was freezing. Then I was called into hair and make-up, where I met Jason Lewis, who played Smith, Samantha's on-screen boyfriend, and my co-star Gilles Marini, who played Dante, Sam and Smith's neighbour in Malibu. Gilles was a smokin' hot French guy, and though I was supposed to be acting I wanted to fuck him for real!

My hair looked fabulous, but they asked for natural

make-up, which is one thing I hate about mainstream shows. I don't feel sexy at all having almost no make-up on, so I sneaked a little more on, since I had brought my own with me. I didn't add too much, though, because I knew they'd get pissed. Then I had to fill in my paper-work and – damn! – that was when I realised I was going to earn three times more than I would for a real sex scene, and all I had to do was a simulated sex scene! God, I love the Screen Actors Guild (SAG). I wish we had the same kind of union in porn. We don't get paid nearly enough money for risking our health and our lives.

I didn't get my wish to fuck Gilles, of course, though I will reveal here that he wasn't wearing a sock, meaning both of us were totally naked. As a mainstream actor, his name wasn't yet known to many people, but after *Sex and the City* came out he called me to say he was getting lots of offers for various things, and I was so happy for him.

Our scene happens about half an hour into the movie, when Samantha, played by Kim Cattrall, is in the jacuzzi and suddenly realises from hearing my moaning and groaning that she has a hot new neighbour – meaning Gilles, not me. (I was playing second fiddle to her second fiddle, so to speak.) It was a funny scene to do because they asked me to moan loudly, over and over again. The idea was to show that I could be heard next door, over the ocean and the double-glazed windows, which in reality would've been impossible. But I think it made it that much funnier, since all you hear is me moaning really loud and then Samantha turning around because she heard me. (I wonder if I turned her on, too. I guess I'll never know.)

In December 2008, I was offered another role in a mainstream show, and this time it was the lead! It was in a HBO film for cable TV, and it was on the condition that I use my real name. While I was debating whether or not to take the plunge and do that, I found out that they couldn't change the shoot dates and I was left with a scheduling conflict – I had to fly out to Tampa Bay in Florida for three days of dance gigs that same week. The HBO people said they couldn't work around my dates, so I lost the part.

At the time, the choice wasn't all that difficult, given the challenging economic climate. Florida was the sure thing, cash in the bank, whereas the movie was a maybe. Then, I was offered another dance gig, in Puerto Rico, and yet another lead role in a mainstream movie came my way. I had to ask myself, 'Should I take the dance gigs with the big money or the cable-TV roles with not as much money but which might help extend my mainstream acting career?'

There was surely no better time for me to rethink my longevity in the adult industry, and I began to reach the conclusion that it was time for a change. They say that change is a good thing if it's the right change, don't they? And if it's the wrong change, well, you're screwed. And I think I'm going to discover which one I'm headed for real soon.

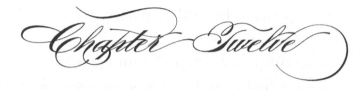

I STILL CALL
AUSTRALIA HOME

I t's been over nine years since I left Australia, but every now and then something will give me a huge pang of homesickness. Recently, I was listening to Soundscapes, the relaxation music station on cable, when suddenly I was in a trance to this awesome Aboriginal music. It made me miss home immensely, where it is so spiritual and beautiful. I missed watching the lightning and thunderstorms in the middle of a hot summer.

You don't realise how great a country Australia is until you leave and see how the rest of the world lives. Especially America. As grateful as I am to be here living the dream in Hollywood, this country does things quite differently, in many ways. Maybe I'm just very patriotic, I don't know, but I still call Australia home. (Poor Peter Allen must be rolling in his grave; I'm sure he never thought he'd ever hear a porn chick say those words – though I suspect that, like most gay men, he surely loved porn stars!)

I'm certainly nostalgic and want to go back, for sure. Of course, I could never have made a career out of porn back home, so it has been a good stay for me, out here in Southern California.

My remaining immediate family still lives in Australia. I'm now quite close to my dad and his wife. They visited me in LA last Christmas and, the year before that, I went to Sydney and spent the holidays with them. They are such good people and they know I love them, even though I know they've been put through quite a lot because of me. For a long time, they never knew what I really did.

When I wrote to my father and told him I was a porn star, to say that he was freaked out would be an under-statement. He sent me a screaming reply in red letters. Then he didn't talk to me for four months. I finally responded by telling him, 'It's my life. I'm not hurting anyone and I'm not pregnant or anything,' or words to that effect. This seemed to eventually sink in and he started talking to me again.

As far as anyone else back home knowing about me, my brother always told anyone who asked that I was living in Los Angeles and I was an actress and a model. My brother is pretty cool with my career – he even came to the AVN Awards in Las Vegas in 2007 and hung out when I was doing my promotional appearances and made funny faces at me when I was signing autographs at the booth. My brother and I have been through a lot. Despite all the bad things he and I experienced while we were growing up, and as much as we both used to fight one another, he would always make me laugh. He still does, to this day. He is just hilarious. So I guess our mother didn't ruin our sense of humour.

Maybe being a smartass was his way of dealing with things, always making a joke out of everything. We used to laugh at our mother whenever she was obviously drunk and we'd say things like, 'Mum's bumping into things again!' She would get so wasted that we'd hear her crashing into the walls in the middle of the night. We still joke about that. At least I have one person in the family who's comfortable with my job, which is more than some porn stars have – a lot of them have fallen out completely with their families because of what they do and aren't on speaking terms any more.

But my career is here now, and when I move more into mainstream movies and music, LA will definitely be the right place to be. After *Sex and the City*, I'm hoping to get into mainstream a little more. I realise that I'll be typecast, but that doesn't bother me. I love acting, and with my SAG card it will be much easier, since the money is fantastic, and it's totally worthwhile being on-set for up to 12 hours a day.

These days I put loads of time and effort into my website, which allows me to work from home more. For a few years, I was signed up with some webmasters who didn't do a good job – not doing enough to generate income from the site and keep my members happy – but after I got out of that contract and went with a different crew things got a lot better. Although, the deal was that my old webmasters would give back the domain name monicamayhemxxx.com and, in return, we'd send them traffic. But, of course, they kept the old site up, still claiming it to be my official site. I've been doing everything I can to put the word out that monicamayhem.com is my real official site. So far, things are going well with the new webmasters; the site is definitely a hundred times better and more personal and interactive with the fans. As for the live chats, I do that for my website members once a month through my own site, and Imlive.com every once in a while, despite the fact that their celebrities only earn 35 per cent. (Seriously, I can be masturbating and talking for two hours, and they get 65 per cent!)

But my life can get pretty lonely sometimes. I'm often home alone, and some nights I just stay in writing songs, watching TV and thinking. I feel like there aren't that many people I can hang out with in LA, because everyone seems so fake here. I have a few real friends, but that's not enough.

I declared that 2008 would be my 'selfish' year. It wasn't totally a success, but I did put my foot down a lot more than I used to. I won't take shit from users any more. No more spending my hard-earned money on other people who are too damn lazy to get a real job. I stopped taking antidepressants, which I had been on for years and which screwed me up even more, made me numb or made me feel like I was going to lose my mind. But I've found that since I've been getting acupuncture and taking Chinese herbs every week, my life has really changed a lot. I may lose motivation or need a change every once in a while, but at least I'm not depressed and miserable any more. I'm pretty sure all the drugs had a big part in why I felt that way for so long.

I still have the asthma, by the way, but it's not nearly as severe as it was. Now, I try to use my inhaler only every other day, because I don't want to have to rely on that to breathe.

I've found it's important to nurture myself when I am at home, so that when I go out into the world I can be at my best. In February 2007 and 2008, for example, I went down to Mexico City for the Mexico Sex & Entertainment show, which is a huge event. In 2008, I was there signing for Kchondiuxx, Pipedream's distributor in Mexico, who paid me and put me up at the W Hotel on Campos Eliseos in Chapultepec Polanco, a very nice area that some people call the Beverly Hills of Mexico City. The city itself is very hectic, very crowded and very noisy, with a lot of traffic. This expo has a ton of fans attending, a ton of entertainment and people announcing stuff very loudly over the speakers nonstop. It's really enough to drive you insane!

I did my own hair and make-up before the show, then sat in a booth surrounded by large posters of myself – not the most flattering picture, but I guess they liked it. The fans had to purchase something before they could get an autograph or take a photo, so it wasn't too hectic that year, and I had a lot of security. When I took a break, there were 50 guys waiting for me, taking my picture as I came out of the toilet. Crazy!

By 8 pm, I was exhausted from eating very little and drinking caffeinated drinks all day. I gave an interview to a guy who made me so mad, questioning why I don't do anal and saying he didn't understand the fact that I don't care that you make more money doing anal. He would not let it go! Then he told me I wasn't a 'real' porn star because of it. I tried to explain to him that it makes no difference, but he then asked what class of porn star I was. I tried to explain that there are no real classes of porn stars, and that 'hardcore' doesn't just mean 'anal'!

Another fan came in for an autograph and photo, and I was so frustrated and offended by this dumbass reporter that I started shaking. I couldn't figure out what was wrong with me. I ate a little, then shut the curtains and lay down. They finally let me leave after five hours of signing. As I was walking out, I thought I was going to fall over. Everything seemed so surreal. I felt like I was on acid. I'm sure the noise, the music and the camera flashes were a big factor as to why I felt this way. I was so scared and didn't want to make too much of a fuss in front of my people.

The organisers don't understand that signing autographs for so long, without a decent break away from the crowds and the noise, is not exactly good for you. I guess I was just wiped out. These ill-informed reporters were there just to toy with me (pardon the pun). Just because I had my own line of vibrators and sex dolls, they treated me with the thinly disguised contempt reserved for women who are little more than whores in their close-minded estimation.

When I got back from Mexico, I decided to kick myself into gear a little more. I signed up with a personal trainer and had my first session. My body-fat percentage was not bad – 24 per cent. I weighed 58 kg and measured 36–28–36. (Wow. I thought I was 34–24–34. I guess I'm a little more curvy now!) The girl training me was a hot Latina, with long black hair and crystal blue eyes. She could be a huge porn star. But I just told her I was a regular actress. I don't like people judging me so I don't tell everyone.

It's a challenge to stay in shape because at this point in my life I feel like I'm permanently on the road. Since I've been shooting fewer porn films, I've been doing more feature dancing, all across the good ol' US of A, often in the most obscure of towns, stuck in the middle of nowhere. A lot of my evenings involve me performing various kinds of uniquely sexy routines. Like my lotion show, called 'Stick It to Monica', where I rub lotion all over my body and then walk around the tip rail to let the guys (and/or girls) stick their dollar bills anywhere they want to! For obvious reasons, this show tends to be the most popular – I mean, who wouldn't want to touch the body of a hot porn star?

Another show I love doing is the paint show, where I take a big piece of canvas that I've pre-signed and kissed and then have the DJ put on the black lights while I daub my body with glow-in-the-dark paints. I'll rub my breasts and my pussy onto the canvas, and – *voila!* – a work of art, which is then auctioned off on stage!

There are a couple of other shows I also like doing. There's one called 'Cooter Ball', where I grip a shot glass between my legs and each guy in the audience has to roll up a dollar bill and try to throw it into the glass. The glass is really small so it's not easy to make the shot. The prize is a DVD, personally signed by me. (If someone gets it in too soon, I'll keep the game going and give another movie away to the next lucky winner.) The other fun show is 'Rides for Five', in which the customers have to lie on their backs onstage, holding up their $5 bills for me, and I go around and give them lap dances, just quick ones but usually sticking my crotch in their faces. In fully nude places, this means that they get my *bare* crotch right up close and personal!

I also love to mess with girls onstage. I'll go up to any women who are sitting at the tip rail (customers or performers – you're fair game if you're at the tip rail) and start slapping their boobs or grabbing them, and they never seem to mind. Often, the strippers will come up onstage just to play with me. I always go around sticking my own tits in everyone's faces (everyone who has at least $1 for me, that is). And, of course, at the end of the show I'll throw out free posters for the fans, who can come up to me and get them signed later. (After every show, I'll be at a signing area, where the fans can come up for a meet-and-greet with me.) I sell them posters, Polaroids, DVDs and magazines. And lap dances, too – for US$100 a song, usually. Most of the time, I meet some pretty cool fans and I'll also get the occasional diehard fan who knows everything that I've ever done and will bring a huge array of box-covers, magazines and other stuff for me to sign. (Then, of course, he'll buy anything else that I have to offer!)

My shows are very high-energy, which takes a lot out of me. Dancing, however, is not what it used to be. Times are tough for everyone these days. I used to get paid twice as much per show, and they would buy two return airfares for me so I could bring a roadie (or an assistant), plus I would always get my demands met for a nice hotel (like a Hilton or a Crowne Plaza). Some clubs would send a limo to pick me up from the airport, as well as to and from the club every night, and the ones with the five-star restaurants would provide me with lobster and filet mignon and all the Cristal (as in the Louis Roederer champagne, not meth!) that I could drink.

Nowadays, I sometimes only get one return airfare, and it's not always first class (although, as a lot of people will agree, first class on a lot of domestic American airlines isn't very good anyway), and I don't always get the nicest hotel. Take, for example, my latest trip to Wisconsin. I started off in Milwaukee, in a Hilton-family hotel that was decent enough but with no room service. Then I got driven 45 minutes away to a ghost town called Juneau (population 2200), where they left me for dead in this old, smelly, dirty apartment right next to the club. The club itself was beautiful and brand new, but this apartment was the worst place I've ever been put in. I had three days off before my next set of shows started, and there was absolutely nothing around and nowhere to eat. (To add insult to injury, there were no utensils in the apartment to cook with, either!) I had to have a friend, who lived 50 minutes away, come and drive me everywhere – including the grocery store, so I could at least have some fresh fruit and veggies.

There's always some kind of drama in every club I go to. Usually, it's a bunch of jealous strippers sitting in the dressing room, talking shit about me, thinking that I'm taking all their money (when, really, I'm helping to bring in money by bringing in more customers, because the whole point of a feature dancer is to draw more people in because of her name). I always have my own dressing room, but sometimes it's right next to where these girls are, and it's always the same annoying drama in every club – girls fighting with each other and bitching, 'You hit on my boyfriend!' or 'I only made twenty dollars tonight!' (which makes me think, well, if they weren't in the back complaining so much, maybe they'd make some more money). All of this drives me insane, so I have to block it out by playing music really loud in my dressing room. I love dancing to hard rock and metal. Not everyone loves it but I feel sexy dancing to it, and that's all that matters. I'll never submit to hip hop and rap – I just can't do it. I have no idea how I would dance to that. (That's all they play in some clubs and I go back to my room with the throbbing bass pumping in my head every night.)

My most recent drama on the road, however, was not with the strippers but rather with one of the owners of a certain club. This guy owned the apartment building I was staying in too, and he brought the club manager and two of the waitresses into my living room for a little after-party – while I was trying to sleep in the bedroom. I was absolutely shocked! I couldn't believe they could have such disrespect. (First of all, they were not supposed to have access to the feature dancer's accommodation. And, secondly, how the fuck did they think it would be okay to throw a party in *my* room, at 3.30 am?) I bit my tongue and didn't say anything, because I still had three more shows to finish the next night and I had to get paid. So, on the next night, it was the manager's birthday and out of revenge I dragged him onstage. I sang a nice happy birthday to him, then had two of his favourite girls come up and embarrass the hell out of him – throwing water on him, whipping him and walking him around like a dog in front of the audience. And this guy was big and buff and a bit of a hardass, so it was absolutely hilarious.

And that's how I ended my most recent show at the time of writing this, after doing 20 shows in two weeks. It was straight to the chiropractor for me when I got back home to LA! I always return from feature dancing black and blue, with bruises from the pole, and my neck and back are always out of place. That might also be due to flying all over the country, trying to sleep on planes – near-impossible, given my permanent state of insomnia. (Sleeping is hard enough even when I'm home, and I refuse to take sleeping pills.)

When I'm not on the road dancing, I spend most of my time *preparing* for the dance gigs (when I'm not working on my website, that is). This includes getting my hair and nails done, going tanning, going to the chiropractor, getting acupuncture and facials and massages, buying my movies to sell to my fans (which I first obtain from the producers at a discount) and buying props for dancing, as well as cleaning my costumes and reorganising my suitcases. But I'm also in and out of meetings and auditions, and I'll do interviews on the road on different radio stations.

I have been doing everything I can to take more care of my body in between my gigs and other commitments, and this has been good for my mind too. I am starting to feel more at peace. I am taking more time to do the things that relax me, such as sitting on the beach in Malibu, with the wind in my face and the sun gleaming over the ocean. It feels so good. Looking out at the Pacific Ocean always makes me feel connected to my homeland, Australia. And I know that as long as I keep working and looking after myself as I have been, and take a day off at least once a week, then I will be fine.

I think I'm beginning to figure out ways of dealing with every situation that comes my way, and how to maintain some sort of balance, instead of relying on the usual 'running in every direction' approach to things – the typical Pisces trait. I know I'll never be perfect, but at least I see my own flaws and I make positive steps to try to change. And I have changed, so much. And I'm still changing.

I'm not miserable or negative all the time, though when I read through old diaries or look at my song lyrics it certainly looks that way. I'm actually a very optimistic person, but when I'm happy I don't usually write down my thoughts. I write more for therapy, to let it out without boring other people with my problems – like most people tend to do to me, because I'm a good listener. Maybe I should start writing my positive thoughts, so I can look back and not feel so bad.

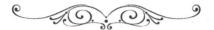

Back in September 2004, I wrote some lyrics in my journal after a horrible dance gig in Pittsburgh. The club owners were extremely rude and treated me so badly that I retaliated by trashing my dressing room like a deranged rock star. I shocked the hell out of my roadie, but I was drunk and pissed off and pleased. Served those idiots right!

So I wrote to calm myself down. I never finished the song, but I still like some of the lyrics. The verses speak volumes for where I was in my life back then:

> Looking at the world though the corner of my eye,
> Time just standing still and I can't explain why.
> I know it's all my fault, I could push harder each day.
> I'm getting closer now, I know I'll find a way . . .
> How can I love myself when everybody loves to hate me?
> They don't see all the pain that I can't seem to set free.
> My foolish eyes, they never lie,
> Except for the scared little girl inside.

And it ends like this, a final refrain:

Turn around, wake up to yourself,
Stop wishing that you were somebody else.

I think about that last bit a lot. True to my chosen name, I've caused a little mayhem for the past eight or nine years. And I know that now, all the characters I've played have come back to only one: me. The only person I'll ever want to be.

Well, in theory, anyway. In reality, I face the mirror every day and wonder.

I guess that's one reason why, of the 400-something movies I've made, the ones I like the most always have to do with how I really see myself, and how I see porn as part of my life.

Looking back over my porn career, it hasn't been all bad. I have had a hell of a lot of good times in this business, and met a lot of very cool people. The single best thing that porn has done for me is boost my self-confidence. I had been hiding behind a wall, protected by the corporate uniform – in the era that began with me working at Westpac and ending at Salomon Smith Barney – and the best way to deal with that was to literally take off that uniform.

I decided to go all the way and take all my clothes off, so that I had nothing left to hide. I had only my own naked body to work with and I learned to express myself that way. And I found I could do much more than I'd anticipated or expected.

When you've spent most of your life being put down by other people, that's not an easy transition at all. But I did all I could, with a little help along the way.

Anyway, before I sign off and fade to black (insert Kirk Hammett guitar riff here, please), here's something that happened to me that puts everything in perspective.

One evening in September 2008, I was at the Kevin Josephson hair salon in Beverly Hills, getting all dolled up – along with the supermodel/TV host Janice Dickinson and a bunch of models from her agency. I did this after I'd been asked if I wanted a free spray-tan and hair-do session in exchange for modelling for that salon and I thought it would be a lark. Anyway, they did the most amazing treatment on my hair – afterwards, it felt so soft and silky, and they touched-up my roots, too. The whole salon was like a zoo, with an open bar and DJ and models and people just coming in to hang out all night.

The spray-tan bit took forever and the stuff took hours to dry. I had to model with no make-up on in front of everyone and with some of Janice's models as well, wearing only a skimpy gold thong bikini.

It was a very long night and I finally left the salon at 12.30 am, after having arrived at 5.30 pm. I'd had no dinner and I was starving, so I pulled over into a McDonald's on the way home. The McDonald's security guard told me he was hungry too, because they wouldn't let him walk through the drive-in area, so I ended up buying the guy some fries.

'There you go, mate. Mind your cholesterol,' I thought, proud of my own display of compassion. This is America, not Africa, but you can find people starving anywhere. Just when you think you're feeling sorry for yourself, you'll discover someone more miserable than you.

And here's the kicker: the thing that nobody knew – not the people at the hair salon and not the security guard – was that I was a porn star who was a nervous wreck inside. Because the very next day I would be getting my latest test results back. And, as usual, I had absolutely no idea if I'd caught anything from anyone or not.

That's my reality, hidden from public view. I freak out silently, once every month.

All of us porn stars do. And no camera can ever capture that.

So, as a Wiccan, all I can ever do is thank the gods and goddesses for every day I'm still alive.

When you're a porn star, you have to be mindful of how you're a professional sex object, like a stripper performing behind a glass panel for guys jerking off on the other side. This is what you're there for, to provide a form of entertainment in the form of sexual release. If you can't deal with that, you should find yourself another career.

That said, it's a complicated thing, trying to get to the bottom of it. I'm sure some people out there think I must have had sex with at least a thousand people by now, but I don't think I've hit that kind of target at all, because I've rotated a lot of the talent – I've worked with many of the same guys over and over and some girls over and over, so I couldn't say how many people I've had sex with. It's definitely more than most people who aren't porn stars can claim – though, as with many things in life, more is not necessarily better.

Being treated as a sex symbol does have its perks, and there are actually a lot of things that I can't complain about. I've been inducted into the Hall of Fame at the Erotic Museum in Las Vegas. I won the 'Golden Throat' trophy at the Sexopolis Sunset Strip Awards held at the Viper Room in Los Angeles in September 2008. And I've been paid to host private house parties and events in swanky nightclubs. In July 2008, I attended a party jointly organised by two porn companies and went with a girl who was new in the business, Sammi Ross. She was like, 'Wow, everyone knows you!' There were so many pornorazzi there and the camera flashes were stunning to her. Everyone always makes me feel like such a big celebrity, and I love that.

It is a bit crazy, though, when these people start pulling me in every direction. When I was leaving, someone dragged me over to meet some famous hip-hop artists. These guys were like, 'Oh yeah, dawg, I seen your movies!' They were all over me and it was hilarious because I've never heard their music, even though I've heard of them. One of them tried to get my phone number but I gave him my email address instead.

Porn stardom is certainly the most unusual form of celebrity that exists in our consumer culture, aside from, perhaps, circus freaks and serial killers (and some people are cynical enough to lump us into the same unfortunate category), and I can assure anyone pondering the state of my own mental health that I am perfectly fine.

I just like being paid to be a professional sex object. I do feel like I am a commodity and I know I am selling my body to make possible the pleasure of others, so I'm never embarrassed about signing autographs for the fans. 'All my luv and sex!' and 'Keep it hard for me!' are what I generally like to write when I'm signing box-covers, which is pretty tame compared to some of the things some of the other girls will write. I see no need to be too nasty on paper, since they're going to be seeing me in the movie anyway and can think every nasty thought of me then.

Honestly, I am proud of the fact that I made a fateful decision to live, as they say, a life less ordinary. I get to choose my lifestyle and work in an industry that many women secretly wish they could be a part of somehow but fear to admit it, much less act on it, because of societal disapproval.

I'm a perfect example of what can happen if you just take a chance and do things on the spur of the moment. You never know how far that might take you.

When I left the corporate world, all I wanted was to be free, to be my own boss, to not have to worry too much about the business side of things, to just be an actress/model and enjoy life. What I've since learned, often the hard way, is that you need a business plan in order to develop your career. There were times when I realised too late that I should have accepted certain contracts being offered to me, and there were certain times in my career when I should have done more mainstream publicity.

And, I'll willingly admit, times when I shouldn't have blown so much money on things I didn't really need – like a very cool car that I really spent a fortune on, getting it all souped up only to lose it, thanks to a wacky quirk of fate called a divorce – and, of course, there were drugs I shouldn't have done and loser 'friends' that I shouldn't have taken care of.

How many more years in porn do I have? I don't know. I never plan ahead like that, because I just go with the flow. I think I will know when it's time to stop. Right now, I can see myself doing this for at least a few more years. Retirement isn't an option yet, though it crosses my mind every now and then.

Whatever happens, I'll always have my website, anyway. Sometimes, like a lot of people, I wish that someone would come and save me and take me away from all my problems. I hope I'll be married again some day. I used to think about the possibility of directing or producing or working behind the camera, but I've decided that's really not my passion. I hate putting my energy into things that I'm not 100-per cent passionate about.

And, of course, I want to be a rock star, after I've done my duty being a porn star. It's a different way of making people happy, and who's to say one is better or one is wrong? I'd rather do both, and discover the truth for myself.

All My Luv & Sex!
♡ Monica Mayhem
xxx

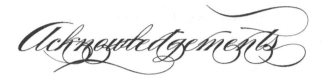

Acknowledgements

*W*e would both like to thank our wonderful team at Ebury Press/Random House – Alison Urquhart (our publisher), Kevin O'Brien and Jessica Dettmann (our editors) and Alysha Farry (our publicist) – who collectively inspired us and kept the faith. (Alison told us she'd read our entire original manuscript over the Christmas holidays in December 2008 in one sitting. We are so not worthy!)

We are also indebted to certain friends for certain things (including drugs and sex . . . just kidding): Jay Allan, Robbye Bentley, Edwina Blush, Sharon Bradley, Annalisa Buoro, Asia Carrera, Dana Duncan Seil, Janiss Garza, Tanya de Grunwald, Chris King, Hank Londoner,

Dee McLaughlin, Jay Moyes, Suze Randall, Brenda Scofield, Joanita Titan, Jeff Wozniak and Sherry Ziegelmeyer.

Special thanks to Alaura Eden and Dez Ballard (in Orange County), Troy (in Maryland) and Kelly Holland (for first introducing us to each other, back when she was still Toni English).

Monica gives big hugs to Rick Bottari, for being her good Aussie mate living in LA and for coming up with the brilliant title *Absolute Mayhem*. She would like to say to Gerrie, 'Without you, this book may not have been made possible. And thanks for being such a great friend!'

Gerrie says the pleasure is mutual and cheers to Smokey. And love always (once more, with feeling) to P. H.

Made in United States
Orlando, FL
20 April 2024